Mayo Clinic on
Healthy Weight

Donald D. Hensrud, M.D.

Editor-in-Chief

MASON CREST PUBLISHERS

Philadelphia, Pennsylvania

Mayo Clinic on Healthy Weight provides reliable, practical, easy-to-understand information on weight management. Much of this information comes directly from the experience of physician nutrition specialists, registered dietitians, and other health care professionals at Mayo Clinic. This book supplements the advice of your physician, whom you should consult for individual medical problems. *Mayo Clinic on Healthy Weight* does not endorse any company or product. MAYO, MAYO CLINIC, MAYO CLINIC HEALTH INFORMATION and the Mayo triple-shield logo are marks of Mayo Foundation for Medical Education and Research.

Hardcover Library Edition Published 2002
Mason Crest Publishers
370 Reed Road
Suite 302
Broomall, PA 19008-0914
(866) MCP-BOOK (toll free)

First printing

1 2 3 4 5 6 7 8 9 10

Library of Congress Cataloging-in-Publication Data on file at the Library of Congress

ISBN 1-59084-225-1

Special thanks to the University of Alabama at Birmingham and to Pennsylvania State University for pioneering work in energy density and weight management. Photographs and recipes in the "Color guide to healthy eating" © *The Mayo Clinic/Williams-Sonoma Cookbook,* Weldon Owen, Inc.

Printed in the United States of America

About healthy weight

More than half of American adults weigh too much. And it's not just a cosmetic issue. Excess weight can harm your health and the quality of your life. The total costs attributable to obesity-related health conditions, some life-threatening, are approaching $100 billion annually.

Every year Americans spend tens of billions of dollars on weight-loss products and services. Some of the plans work. Many fail to provide lasting results.

This book offers a new Mayo Clinic approach to the achievement of healthy weight. Much of the information is what Mayo Clinic doctors and dietitians use day in and day out in caring for people who come seeking assistance with weight control.

If you put the information in this book to work in your daily living, you'll achieve and maintain the weight that's right, and healthiest, for you.

About Mayo Clinic

Mayo Clinic evolved from the frontier practice of Dr. William Worrall Mayo, and the partnership of his two sons, William J. and Charles H. Mayo, in the early 1900s. Pressed by the demands of their busy surgical practice in Rochester, Minn., the Mayo brothers invited other physicians to join them, pioneering the private group practice of medicine. Today, with more than 2,000 physicians and scientists at its three major locations in Rochester, Minn., Jacksonville, Fla., and Scottsdale, Ariz., Mayo Clinic is dedicated to providing comprehensive diagnoses, accurate answers and effective treatments.

With its depth of knowledge, experience and expertise, Mayo Clinic occupies an unparalleled position as a health information resource. Since 1983, Mayo Clinic has published reliable health information for millions of consumers through award-winning newsletters, books and online services. Revenue from the publishing activities supports Mayo Clinic programs, including medical education and research.

Editorial staff

Editor in Chief
Donald D. Hensrud, M.D.

Managing Editor
David E. Swanson

Copy Editor
Edith Schwager

Editorial Researchers
Deirdre A. Herman
Shawna L. O'Reilly

Contributing Writers
Linda Kephart Flynn
Michael J. Flynn
Stephen M. Miller
Robin Silverman
Christina Verni

Creative Director
Daniel W. Brevick

Graphic Designer
Stewart J. Koski

Medical Illustrator
John V. Hagen

Photographers
Joseph M. Kane
Richard D. Madsen
Randy J. Ziegler

Editorial Assistant
Carol A. Olson

Indexer
Larry Harrison

Reviewers and additional contributors

Haitham S. Abu-Lebdeh, M.D.
Matthew M. Clark, Ph.D.
Maria Collazo-Clavel, M.D.
Mark Glen, R.D.
Daniel L. Hurley, M.D.
Michael D. Jensen, M.D.
Frank P. Kennedy, M.D.
James A. Levine, M.D.
M. Molly McMahon, M.D.
Michael A. Morrey, Ph.D.
Jennifer K. Nelson, R.D.
Timothy O'Brien, M.D.
Michael G. Sarr, M.D.

Preface

I'm going to make an assumption. You wouldn't be holding this book if you were not concerned about your weight. The solution to weight management sounds easy — eat less and exercise more. But putting this into practice can be more challenging than it sounds.

You've probably tried to lose weight, perhaps with limited success. You're in good company. Most adult Americans need to trim down; some need to lose a great deal of weight. Either way, there's no shortage of plans. The bookstores, television channels and Internet are filled with products, plans and services.

You won't find The Mayo Clinic Diet in this book because it doesn't exist (see page 103). But we do introduce our new Mayo Clinic Healthy Weight Pyramid™, which is vital to our approach to permanent weight management. And you will find all the easy-to-understand information you need to determine the weight that's right for you, and to achieve and maintain that weight for the rest of your life. You'll also discover helpful links to our Web site, *MayoClinic.com*, our online source for reliable health information.

If you act on the information in this book, there will be short- and long-term effects. You'll begin to feel better immediately. Most important, there will be substantial health benefits. You'll reduce your risk of serious, weight-related illnesses.

Making beneficial lifestyle changes in the way you eat and in your physical activity are keys to healthy weight. But this doesn't have to be drudgery. The lifestyle that leads to permanent healthy weight should be and can be an enjoyable way to live.

Donald D. Hensrud, M.D.
Editor in Chief

Contents

Preface   v

Part 1: Getting motivated

Chapter 1 **Where to start**   3
             The unhealthy truth   4
             The bulking of America   5
             The joy of success   6
             Blame and shame   8
             Calories, not volume   9
             On your way   12

Chapter 2 **Are you too heavy?**   15
             What is obesity?   15
             What's your BMI?   16
             Tale of the tape   18

Chapter 3 **What causes obesity?**   21
             Your genes   21
             Your diet   22
             Your activity   23
             Understanding weight control   26
             The good news   28

Chapter 4 **Is your health at risk?**   29
             Avoidable health problems   29
             Can your weight affect your life span?   33
             Self-assessment tools   33
             Do you really need to lose weight?   36

Chapter 5	**Measuring the challenge**	39
	Identifying your unique challenges	40
	Preparing to change	42
	Starting with a commitment	43
	Setting goals	45
	Planning ahead	46
Chapter 6	**Fundamentals of healthy eating**	49
	Variety is the spice of life	50
	Calories do count	52
	Fat in your diet	52
	Carbohydrates in your diet	55
	Watch those portion sizes	57
	Energy density — Feeling full on fewer calories	58
	Food group fundamentals	59
	Shrewd shopping	64
	Preparing healthy foods	67
	Eating out	72

Part 2: How to lose weight

Chapter 7	**Converting knowledge to action**	77
	A new approach to healthy weight	77
	Daily dining record	92
	Putting our pyramid approach to work for you	94
	Daily menus	94
	Advanced menu planning	102
COLOR SECTION	**Color guide to healthy eating**	C1
	Mayo Clinic Healthy Weight Pyramid	C2
	How many daily servings?	C4
	Our best-of-the-best food recommendations	C4
	What's a serving?	C5
	Recipe section	C7-C16

Chapter 8	**Physical activity**	105
	Weighing the merits	106
	Tailoring your personal program	107
	The family way	111
	Taking the next step	113
	Crafting a plan	115
	Aerobic exercise	116
	Strength and balance	120
	Flexibility and stretching	121
	Recording your progress	122
	A new attitude	124
Chapter 9	**Changing attitudes and actions**	125
	First, think this through	126
	Know thyself	129
	How to change	130
	Deprivation is a no-no	138
	Accentuate the positive	139
	Time is on your side	140
	Put your whole self in	142
Chapter 10	**When the going gets tough**	145
	Forming good habits	146
	Get real	149
	A solution for every problem	151
	Willpower vs. self-control	153
	Friends in need	156
	Staying the course	157
	And finally ...	160
Chapter 11	**Other eating plans**	161
	Low-calorie liquid diets	162
	Low-calorie solid-food diets	163
	Fad diets	165
	Prepared-food diets	168
	Commercial group approaches	169
	Now's the time	172

Part 3: When you need more help

Chapter 12 **Medications for weight loss** 175

Who's a candidate? 176

Popular prescription medications 178

Popular over-the-counter drugs 180

Chapter 13 **Surgery for weight loss** 185

Is surgery right for you? 186

How your digestive system works 187

Options to consider 188

Side effects of surgery 192

Making the adjustments 193

It takes more than surgery 194

Appendix **Recipes you can rely on** 195

Sunshine juice blend 196

Provencal chicken and fennel 196

Summer savory spinach frittata 197

Wild rice-and-chicken salad 198

Thai-style mushroom-and-tofu stir-fry 199

Gingered carrot soup 199

Index 201

Part 1

Getting motivated

Chapter 1
Where to start   3

- The unhealthy truth   4
- The bulking of America   5
- The joy of success   6
- Blame and shame   8
- Calories, not volume   9
- On your way   12

Chapter 2
Are you too heavy?   15

- What is obesity?   15
- What's your BMI?   16
- Tale of the tape   18

Chapter 3
What causes obesity?   21

- Your genes   21
- Your diet   22
- Your activity   23
- Understanding weight control   26
- The good news   28

Chapter 4
Is your health at risk?   29

- Avoidable health problems 29
- Can your weight affect your life span?   33
- Self-assessment tools   33
- Do you really need to lose weight?   36

Chapter 5
Measuring the challenge   39

- Identifying your unique challenges   40
- Preparing to change   42
- Starting with a commitment   43
- Setting goals   45
- Planning ahead   46

Chapter 6
Fundamentals of healthy eating   49

- Variety is the spice of life   50
- Calories do count   52
- Fat in your diet   52
- Carbohydrates in your diet   55
- Watch those portion sizes   57
- Energy density — feeling full on fewer calories   58
- Food group fundamentals 59
- Shrewd shopping   64
- Preparing healthy foods   67
- Eating out   72

Chapter 1

Where to start

Take-home messages

- Before you start, make sure you're ready for the journey. It will be rewarding.
- Your health will improve if you lose excess pounds.
- You can shed weight by establishing healthy habits.
- Your diet and level of physical activity are keys to healthy weight.
- Managing weight is challenging but not impossible. It starts with attitude.
- Make a commitment to a sustained lifestyle change.
- Be sure your new lifestyle is pleasant and enjoyable.
- Consistency, not perfection, is the key to success.

If you're like 97 million other Americans, you weigh more than you should. Let's face it — in this culture, it's easy to pack on pounds, what with the availability of calorie-dense foods, the bombardment of commercial messages urging you to eat, supersized portions and labor-saving devices that keep you from moving.

The human body wasn't designed to overeat high-fat, processed foods, then sit in front of a computer or TV screen much of the day. It was, however, designed to store fat so that our ancestors wouldn't starve when they couldn't find food. That's the job of your body's 30 billion to 40 billion fat cells. Poor things. They don't know that times have changed. Combine your body's propensity for storing fat with today's inactive, high-calorie-consuming lifestyles, and you may feel as though you're doomed to be overweight. You're not. You have choices.

But how to get motivated? You've heard over and over that

losing weight is beneficial. But even if you really want to lose weight, there are so many confusing messages about how to do it, it's hard to know where to turn.

Low fat. High fat. A lot of protein. Not much protein. Carbohydrate loading. Restricting carbs. Different diets promote different eating plans. They can't all be right. What's best for you?

Maybe you've tried and failed in the past, perhaps many times, either because you didn't lose weight or because you lost and regained it. Maybe you can't stomach the thought of one more eating plan. Is it worth it to try again, you wonder. How would this time be different? And, really, you ask, what's so bad about being overweight?

The unhealthy truth

Here's what's so bad: You could be risking your health, especially if you're both overweight and physically unfit. It's even worse if you carry your weight around your middle (apple shape) rather than in your buttocks, hips and thighs (pear shape). Why? Because fat around your middle is even more strongly associated with serious health risks.

As you get older, your potential for developing health problems as a result of being overweight increases. You've undoubtedly heard the litany before, but it bears repeating. Being overweight puts you at greater risk of developing:

- High blood pressure
- Abnormal levels of blood fats (high triglycerides and low HDL "good" cholesterol)
- Type 2 diabetes mellitus
- Coronary artery disease
- Stroke
- Gallbladder disease
- Osteoarthritis
- Respiratory problems (sleep apnea)
- Certain types of cancer (uterine, gallbladder, colon and breast cancer in women, and colon and prostate cancer in men)

All of these problems can shorten your life; any will interfere with the quality of your life (see pages 29-33).

The good news is that even a small weight loss, 5 percent to 10 percent of your current weight, will lower your health risks. A small weight loss may help lower your blood pressure, improve your blood fat levels, reduce sleep apnea symptoms and bring your diabetes under better control. But if you're not experiencing health problems now, then chances are the threat of them in the future is not a strong motivator for you, even if it should be. What about the impact of your weight on your day-to-day life? How's your energy level? What about your self-esteem? Your mood? Your outlook on life?

Maybe you've felt the sting of judgment from others because of your weight. It's ironic that in a culture where so many people are overweight, some discriminate against the obese. If you've ever missed out on a job opportunity because of your weight, been laughed at, or had someone ask you on a crowded airplane why you didn't pay for two seats, you know how much it hurts. Perhaps a little personal success in the weight-control department could give you a boost.

Improving your health over the long haul is the most important reason for reaching and maintaining a healthy weight. But, along the way, feeling better physically, feeling better about yourself and, perhaps, looking better, aren't bad short-term payoffs for taking on a tough challenge. They may even spur you on to reach your long-term goal.

The bulking of America

Overweight and obesity (severe overweight) have become a national epidemic. An estimated 55 percent of adult Americans are obese or overweight. And if that's not enough, the number of people who are obese has increased by more than one-third in the last 20 years. It's a growing problem in more ways than one, and the only entity profiting is the diet industry. Americans spend more than $34 billion a year for weight-loss products and services. In far too many cases, they get no long-term benefit for their investment.

With all that money spent on solutions, you'd think more people would succeed at losing weight. Part of the problem is that people try to lose weight for the wrong reasons, such as dropping from a size 14 to a size 6 in time for a high school reunion or achieving the cultural standards of beauty set by actors and supermodels. Of course, your appearance is important, but beauty is subjective, and few of us look like models. It's your health that really matters.

Another problem is that weight management is hard. It's understandable that you want an easy, quick fix. But overweight and obesity are complex problems, complicated by genes, environment and emotional issues. You probably didn't gain the extra weight quickly, yet you want it gone now. So maybe you try the latest diet or the hottest diet supplement. You lose weight. You feel inspired.

Chances are, though, that unless you made long-term lifestyle changes to alter your eating habits in sustainable ways and became more physically active, the pounds came back on, perhaps bringing a few extra with them. And now you're even more convinced than ever that you can't succeed.

Yes, you can.

The joy of success

Undoubtedly you think that pursuing healthy weight has to be a bore. You've been on diets before. They're all about restrictions, deprivation, food that tastes like cardboard and hours of tedious exercise, aren't they?

It doesn't have to be that way.

Adapting healthy behaviors can be pleasurable. Nutritious food can taste wonderful. Most important, you can change. You can even change your taste buds, believe it or not. If your favorite meal comprises a cheeseburger, fries and a thick chocolate malt, then you need to understand that your taste buds hum when all that salt, fat and sugar hits them because that's what you've trained them to do. It's never too late to teach old buds new tricks.

Even though reaching and maintaining a healthy weight can be a positive experience, that doesn't mean it's easy. There's no magic bullet. No matter how much you hear about the latest herbal diet supplement or the trendy low-carbohydrate diets, no matter how much you want to believe that eating foods in certain combinations will speed weight loss, the human body cannot defy the laws of thermodynamics. To lose weight you have to expend more energy than you take in. Put simply: You have to eat fewer calories and move more.

Boring. You've heard that advice before. So what would possibly be different for you if you tried to follow it again now?

For starters: Attitude. You have to cultivate a positive attitude about making lifestyle changes, and that could require some major retooling. Chances are you have a dieter's mentality. Do any of these sound familiar?

- There are good and bad foods.
- I'm either on a diet or off.
- If I eat something I like, then I'm cheating.
- Staying on my diet takes a lot of willpower.
- Being on a diet means always being hungry.
- Being on a diet means I have to deprive myself of my favorite foods.
- If I have a setback, such as skipping my walk or eating something I hadn't planned to eat, then I'm a failure.

Wrong, wrong, wrong. A clerk in a grocery store recently was overheard commenting to some customers that he had been on a diet for months, but that night he was looking forward to making lasagna. The young man was going off his diet, he said, so he could eat something that tasted good.

Not a winning attitude. There are plenty of recipes for great-tasting, healthy lasagna that he could include in his eating plan. Yet in his mind, he can only eat foods he likes if he goes "off" his diet. That attitude sets him up to fail. He's not focusing on the benefits of his weight loss. He's always waiting until his diet is over so he can eat the way he likes, rather than adopting eating habits that enable him to include healthier, lower-calorie, great-tasting versions of his favorite foods and giving his taste buds a chance to change.

Blame and shame

The other side of a dieter's attitude is blame. "I'm overweight because my mom is." "It's my spouse's cooking." "I don't eat much, so there must be something wrong with my metabolism." Here's the truth:

- Genetics certainly play a part in how your body handles calories. A family history of obesity increases your chances of becoming obese by about 25 to 30 percent. But there's more to life than heredity. You're not doomed. Chances are, along with your mom's tendency to be overweight, she passed on some unhealthy habits that contribute to your problem. You can change those. You'll probably never be able to consume the amount of food your lean and active friend does, but that doesn't mean you can't reach and maintain a healthy weight. Yes, you have to work harder, but you can succeed. This falls in the "life isn't fair" category. To succeed, you'll have to get over feelings of being cheated or doomed to failure.

- Muscle uses more energy than fat does, so men, who have more muscle naturally, burn between 10 percent and 20 percent more calories than women even at rest. So for women, achieving healthy weight may be a tougher challenge. It's still achievable, and well worth doing.

- As you get older, you tend to lose some of that precious calorie-burning muscle, and your percentage of body fat increases. As a result, your metabolism slows slightly. But research has shown that strength training can help burn more calories at rest by maintaining muscle mass. Strength training also offers a host of other benefits, including increasing your ability to perform everyday tasks, improving your balance and decreasing your risk of osteoporosis.

- Sorry, but less than 2 percent of those who are obese have a metabolic disorder or hormonal imbalance. If you think you have one, then by all means consult your doctor. But don't use it as an excuse. In fact, if you're overweight, chances are your weight is causing your metabolism to be higher, so that you burn more calories at rest than your lean friends.

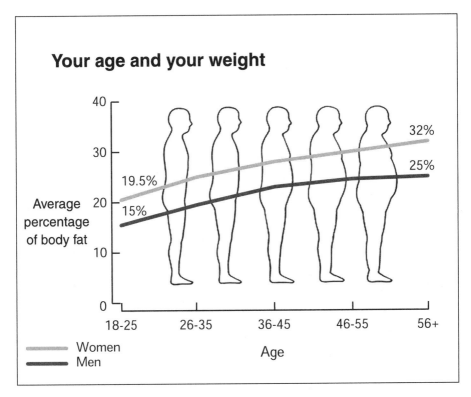

Your age and your weight

Getting older usually means getting fatter. With age, the amount of muscle tends to drop, and fat accounts for a greater percentage of weight.

Calories, not volume

The simplest explanation for why Americans are getting heavier is that we have too many machines that move for us, such as elevators and cars and remote controls, and we eat too many rich foods. But it's not just rich foods, it's unhealthy foods.

In recent years, when fat-reduced foods became the rage, people added extra sugar to make them taste better, and thought they could eat them in unlimited quantities. As a result, people's average yearly sugar intake increased from 127 pounds in 1986 to a whopping 152 pounds in 1996. That's an extra 45,000 calories a year.

Ironically, even with those extra calories, you might still feel hungry. There's evidence that being satisfied may be more strongly determined by the volume and weight of food you consume rather than the number of calories. In other words, fruits, vegetables and other high-fiber foods are bulkier than, say, high-fat foods or refined low-fat foods, so they fill you up better, without the extra calories.

Think about this: You could eat 10 to 15 medium apples, 10 or 11 heads of lettuce or 35 cups of green beans for the same number of calories you'd find in one and one-third sticks of butter or 5

Are you ready to lose weight?

Because losing weight requires a lot of focus and mental and physical energy, you can't just plunge in. You need to make a commitment and prepare yourself. Part of that preparation is determining whether now is the right time. It's OK if it's not. Your success depends on your readiness to take this challenge on. Ask yourself the following:

- *How motivated do I feel to make lifestyle changes now?* Be honest. Knowing you need to make changes and feeling up to the challenge are two different things.
- *What's going on in my life now and over the next several months?* Be aware you may set yourself up for failure by trying to improve your lifestyle if you're distracted by other major problems, whether they involve your marriage, your job, your finances or your kids. Give your life a chance to calm down before you start. Making the lifestyle changes necessary to achieve and maintain your healthy weight needs to be your highest priority.
- *Am I being realistic about my weight-loss goals?* Remember, losing just 5 percent to 10 percent of your body weight can reap health rewards. Start small. Work on losing 5 pounds at a time. Just because you wore a size 6 dress or 28-waist jeans in high school doesn't mean you should now. Try achieving a comfortable weight you maintained easily as a young adult. If you've always been heavy, then aim for a weight that causes your blood pressure, cholesterol levels, energy and sleep to improve.
- *Do I truly believe that slower is better?* You want to aim for a loss of 1 to 2 pounds a week. That can seem agonizingly

chocolate bars (1^1/$_2$ ounce-size). The same is true of many foods that are high not only in fat but also other concentrated calories such as sugar. So if you add up the fat and sugar you eat in a day, not just in butter and chocolate, but in processed foods, dairy products, meats, candy and low-fat products that are high in sugar, then just how much are you eating?

slow in our instant gratification society. But make improving your health your long-term goal, and speed won't matter.

- *Do I have time to keep records about my food intake and physical activity?* Studies show that keeping records increases your chances of success.
- *Do I have family and friends who will support my efforts?* You need to have someone in your corner. The more the merrier. If you don't, then you might consider meeting regularly with a registered dietitian or joining a group weight-loss program.
- *Do I want to improve my health, or am I just interested in looking better?*
- *Do I believe I can change my eating behavior?*
- *Am I willing to find ways to be more physically active?* Moving more is essential to successful weight loss and maintenance.
- *Do I have an eating disorder or other emotional issues I need to get help for before I can do this?* If you have a tendency to binge and purge, or to starve and overexert when you exercise, or if you're depressed or anxious, then you may want to seek professional help.
- *Am I willing to look at my past successes and failures, in weight loss and other areas of my life, to see what motivates me and keeps me working on things that are obstacles to success?*
- *Do I believe that achieving and maintaining healthy weight is a lifelong process that requires me to change my behavior, my eating habits and my level of physical activity, and am I ready to make that commitment?*
- *Can I view this as a positive, even pleasurable, experience?*

Eating high-fat, calorie-laden, sugary foods is a habit you've learned, so you can unlearn it. Most important, you can learn to eat better.

On your way

As you read through this book, we're going to offer you some very practical advice on everything from how to determine your healthy weight to developing an eating and activity plan, to identifying your obstacles toward achieving your goals, to motivating yourself. Think of this book as your personal coach.

You've undoubtedly heard the grim statistics about how few people succeed at losing weight and keeping it off. Forget that. For one thing, despite the statistics, plenty of people succeed. Sure — you're taking on a tough challenge, possibly one of the hardest you'll tackle. But you're not just anyone. With knowledge, the right attitude and a good plan, you can do anything.

The best news is, as you begin to feel better and have more energy, as you discover how good it feels to move your body, as you learn the sheer pleasure of eating food that makes you healthy, you'll realize how enjoyable this process can be. If you focus on your health, then you'll develop healthy habits. If you develop healthy habits, then the pounds will take care of themselves. And even if you don't reach your "ideal" weight, you'll still be much healthier.

Remember, this is not a quick fix. Anything that promises you quick and easy results or tells you you can lose weight without making lifestyle changes is rubbish. Ignore it. If you're serious about achieving and maintaining healthy weight, then pay no heed

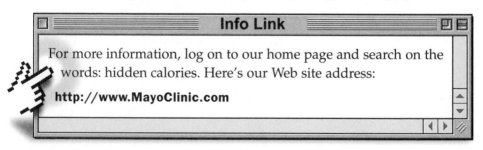

Info Link

For more information, log on to our home page and search on the words: hidden calories. Here's our Web site address:

http://www.MayoClinic.com

Taking control

For about a year before I decided to lose weight, lots of things in my life were out of my control. Losing weight was something I could control.

One of the reasons I could stay with it was that people I worked with and my sister and I decided to do it together. I had a lot of support. That made it fun.

I went to Weight Watchers. I stayed for meetings and kept a food diary. The routine was comforting. It was fun to try new recipes. Another motivator was when people started noticing.

I went out of town for a wedding after I'd been on the program for 2 or 3 weeks. I had considered not starting the program until after the wedding. But I was able to stick with the program, and it didn't affect what kind of time I had.

Shortly after that, I went to Israel for 3 weeks. There it was a little harder to stick with it, but I was aware of what I was eating and doing a lot of walking, so I still lost weight.

By making good food choices and walking for 30 minutes 4 to 5 times a week, I lost 50 pounds in about 11 months. There was a period when my in-laws were in a nursing home. My time for exercise went to visiting them. I served breakfast at the home for four months. Instead of using a cart to carry beverages to the tables, I carried two glasses at a time, back and forth. I told people it was how I got my exercise.

I used to be a stress eater. If I was under stress, I thought chocolate would help. I might still do that, but now I can do with a bite, not a bag. I can have one cookie instead of six. I tell myself, "You don't have to do this."

Now I feel more like I can be in control of things. It's been good for me mentally as well as physically.

Marcia
Overland Park, Kansas

to the fad diets, the herbal supplements, the liquid fasts and the teas or other potions that promise to help you burn calories. Your main concern is your health. And the key to achieving good health is healthy habits.

Now get ready. This is a lifetime commitment to healthy living. Just wait and see how good you're going to feel.

Chapter 2

Are you too heavy?

If you're reading this, chances are you may be too heavy. Before figuring out if you are too heavy by medical standards, remember that most of what you see in the media is not reality. Fashion models and movie stars typically are unrealistically thin, and you should neither expect nor attempt to look like these individuals. Your goal is to attain a healthy weight — one that reduces your risks of disease and health conditions associated with overweight and obesity, and one at which you feel better.

What is obesity?

In simplest terms, obesity is being seriously overweight because of excess body fat. Traditionally, "overweight" has been defined as weighing more than the healthy weight listed in a height-weight table. But that doesn't account for differences in body composition. For example, athletes often are overweight by weight-table standards because of muscle development or a large bone structure. But they are not overfat.

Body fat, instead of weight, is a better predictor of health.

In healthy adults, acceptable levels of body fat range from 18 percent to 23 percent in men and from 25 percent to 30 percent in women. But simply stepping on the scale won't tell you how much of your weight is fat or where you're carrying that fat. Both of these factors are more important in determining health risks than weight alone. The key to body fat analysis is having a trained professional use a reliable method of estimation, such as skinfold measurements or bioelectrical impedance. All methods only give a ballpark figure, however, and the older you are and the more fat you're carrying, the less reliable the measurement may be.

Weight is commonly used to determine health risk because it is much easier to measure than body fat.

What's your BMI?

In 1998, the National Institutes of Health — the federal government's main health research institution — established a new classification system for overweight and obesity based on the body mass index (BMI). The BMI is a formula that is determined by both your weight and height. It is a better estimate of body fat and health risks than your bathroom scale or the standard height and weight tables.

To determine your body mass index, locate your height on the chart on page 17 and follow it across until you reach the weight nearest yours. Look at the top of the table for the BMI rating. A BMI of 18.5 to 24.9 is considered the healthiest. People with a BMI between 25 and 29.9 are considered overweight. People with a BMI of 30 or greater are considered obese.

If your BMI is 25 or greater, shedding pounds may improve your health and reduce your risk of weight-related diseases. If your BMI falls within the healthy range of 19 to 24, there generally is no health advantage for you to lose weight. You can stay within this range by maintaining healthy habits, such as eating a balanced and nutritious diet and engaging in regular physical activity. Reassess your BMI at least every two years and talk to your physician or health care provider if you see significant changes in either direction. If your BMI falls below 19, you're probably underweight.

Ask your doctor to assess your weight and health.

The BMI is a useful tool for monitoring your progress in managing your weight. To calculate your exact BMI so that you can keep track of changes, follow these steps:

Step 1: Multiply your weight in pounds by 0.45

For example, if you weigh 200 pounds: 200 x 0.45 = 90

Step 2: Multiply your height in inches by 0.0254

For example, if you're 5'6" (66 inches): 66 x 0.0254 = 1.68

Step 3: Square the answer from step 2

(1.68 x 1.68 = 2.82)

Step 4: Divide the answer from step 1 by the answer from step 3. This number is your BMI.

(90/2.82 = 32)

(If you're using the metric system, your BMI equals your weight in kilograms divided by the square of your height in meters.)

	HEALTHY		OVERWEIGHT		OBESE			
BMI	19	24	25	29	30	35	40	45
HEIGHT	WEIGHT IN POUNDS							
4'10"	91	115	119	138	143	167	191	215
4'11"	94	119	124	143	148	173	198	222
5'0"	97	123	128	148	153	179	204	230
5'1"	100	127	132	153	158	185	211	238
5'2"	104	131	136	158	164	191	218	246
5'3"	107	135	141	163	169	197	225	254
5'4"	110	140	145	169	174	204	232	262
5'5"	114	144	150	174	180	210	240	270
5'6"	118	148	155	179	186	216	247	278
5'7"	121	153	159	185	191	223	255	287
5'8"	125	158	164	190	197	230	262	295
5'9"	128	162	169	196	203	236	270	304
5'10"	132	167	174	202	209	243	278	313
5'11"	136	172	179	208	215	250	286	322
6'0"	140	177	184	213	221	258	294	331
6'1"	144	182	189	219	227	265	302	340
6'2"	148	186	194	225	233	272	311	350
6'3"	152	192	200	232	240	279	319	359
6'4"	156	197	205	238	246	287	328	369

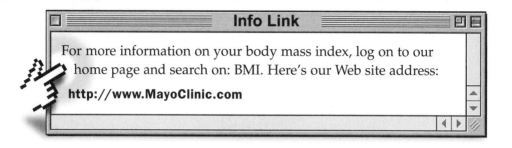

Tale of the tape

Your waist size is another measurement that is useful in determining weight-related health risks. It indicates where most of your fat is located. Fat around your middle is associated with a higher risk of coronary artery disease, high blood pressure, diabetes, stroke and certain types of cancer (see pages 29-33).

To determine whether you're carrying too much weight around your middle, measure your waist. Find the highest point on each hip-bone and measure across your abdomen just above those points. A measurement exceeding 40 inches (102 centimeters) in men or 35 inches (88 centimeters) in women signifies increased health risks. If you have a BMI of 25 or higher, your risk is even greater. Although these cutoffs of 40 and 35 inches are a useful guide, there is nothing magical about them. The bigger the waist, the greater the health risks.

If you have a BMI of 35 or greater, it is likely that your waist measurement will be greater than the cutoff for your sex.

Is your health at risk?

YOUR BMI	YOUR WAIST MEASUREMENTS			
	Female		Male	
	Fewer than 35 inches	35 inches or more	Fewer than 40 inches	40 inches or more
25 to 29.9	Increased	High	Increased	High
30 to 34.9	High	Very high	High	Very high
35 to 39.9	Very high	Very high	Very high	Very high
40 or higher	Extremely high	Extremely high	Extremely high	Extremely high

If your BMI is between 18.5 and 24.9, your health is likely not at risk from your weight. Over 25, you may be at increased risk of serious health complications.

Are you too thin?

BMIs greater than 18.5 and less than 25 are generally considered healthy. Is your BMI lower than 18.5? You may be genetically thin. It could be difficult for you to gain weight without gaining mostly fat. This would not improve your health. Consider these questions:

- Do you have a history of unexplained weight loss? If so, see your doctor — a medical evaluation may be necessary.
- Do you have any medical conditions or are you taking any medications that can cause weight loss?

As in losing weight, gaining weight also requires a combination of diet and exercise. If you need to gain weight, this is how you should start:

- Engage in regular resistance exercise, better known as weight training. This will help you to gain muscle and not fat.
- Choose healthy high-calorie foods such as nuts and seeds and dried fruits. Add nonfat dry milk powder to foods such as skim milk, oatmeal, hot cocoa, tuna or chicken salad and mashed potatoes. Use olive oil or canola oil to cook or add to your foods, or as a base for salad dressings.

Monitor your progress and keep your health care provider informed of changes in your weight and your routine.

Chapter 3

What causes obesity?

Take-home messages

- Genetic factors may influence your likelihood of being obese.
- Your diet and activity ultimately determine your body weight.
- You put on weight when the calories you eat are more than the calories you burn.

In recent years, obesity rates have risen alarmingly in the United States and other developed countries. And the trend is seen in developing countries as they become more industrialized. Increased availability of food — especially calorie-dense foods — coupled with marketing pressures, suboptimal eating habits and sedentary lifestyles significantly contribute to the rise in overweight and obesity that we are seeing in our nation and around the world.

Obesity is a chronic disease that develops from the complex interaction between genes and the environment. Our understanding of how and why obesity develops is incomplete, but it involves a combination of social, behavioral, cultural, physiologic, metabolic and genetic factors.

Your genes

Genes may set the stage for overweight or obesity, but your body weight ultimately is determined by your diet and physical activity. Over the long term, eating excess calories, leading a sedentary lifestyle, or a combination of both leads to obesity.

When you eat more calories than you burn, you gain weight. Although your genes have less influence over your weight than do your behaviors, heredity does play a part in the development of obesity.

But your heredity doesn't mean you're destined to be fat. Your genes can make you more susceptible to weight gain. Your genes affect the rate at which your body accumulates fat and where that fat is stored.

A family history of obesity increases your chance of becoming obese by about 30 percent. Other obesity risk factors, such as what you eat and your activity level, are strongly influenced by your family as well.

So heredity may make it more difficult for you to lose weight than someone whose ancestors were thin. But just as genes don't guarantee cancer or diabetes, they don't decree that you've got to be overweight either. No matter what your genes say, it is ultimately your choices in nutrition and activity that will determine your weight.

Your diet

Americans are eating out more than ever. About 44 cents of every dollar spent on food is for meals eaten away from home. Fast-food restaurants, offering a wide variety of high-calorie, high-fat menu items, are springing up everywhere, and "supersizing" is the norm. Many restaurants, not just fast-food shops, are offering bigger portions in an attempt to attract and compete for customers. But bigger doesn't always mean better. In fact, it usually doesn't.

Even foods eaten in the home — still a significant source of daily calories — often are high in fat and calories as well. Ounce for ounce, fat provides more than twice as many calories as carbohydrate or protein. This energy difference may explain how fat promotes weight gain.

Foods and beverages with a high content of sugar also often contribute to weight gain. Soft drinks, candy and desserts are loaded with empty calories, meaning they provide few, if any, nutrients other than energy. Foods high in fat and sugar are energy dense and may contribute to obesity.

Processed foods (most products other than fresh foods) often have hidden fat and sugar, which are added to improve shelf life, enhance flavor, or both. The ever-increasing flood of new food products into the market, coupled with aggressive, sophisticated marketing practices in the mass media, supermarkets and restaurants, promotes high-calorie consumption. The overall abundance of food in developed countries such as the United States also encourages overeating.

What is a diet?

You've heard the word *diet* all your life, but what does it really mean? And how is it used in this book? Many people use it to imply weight-loss diet. You've heard, or perhaps even said, "No thank you, I'm on a diet." The fact is, anyone who eats food is on a diet. The word *diet* is a general term that simply refers to the foods you eat. Health professionals most often use it in this way. When you see *diet* in this book, it is used to refer to the foods you eat and not intended to imply "weight-loss diet."

Your activity

Physical inactivity characterizes most Americans — more than 60 percent hardly exercise at all. And that's unfortunate. Exercise is effective in warding off obesity, but most Americans are not taking advantage of this preventive approach. Physical exertion has been engineered out of occupations and lifestyles. Automation and other technologies have contributed greatly to lessening physical activity — making it more difficult for you to burn off excess calories. Physical activity must now be more consciously incorporated into daily life because of the conveniences of cars, computers, elevators and other machines.

Overweight people usually are less physically active than normal-weight adults. Whether it's through a structured exercise

routine or just physical activities of daily living, normal-weight
individuals tend to be more active. But inactivity isn't always the
cause of obesity. Lack of exercise may also be the result of being
overweight. Without physical activity you experience a gradual
decline in your ability to perform activities that require physical
effort. You lose strength, endurance and flexibility. Daily activities
gradually become more difficult.

Are you sedentary?
You are sedentary if you:
- Spend most of your day sitting
- Seldom walk more than a block
- Have leisure activities that don't require you to move from
  place to place
- Have a job that keeps you inactive
- Don't take 20 to 30 minutes to exercise at least weekly

For many years, the common belief was that you had to exercise
vigorously if you wanted to become physically fit and improve your
health. As a result, people developed an all-or-nothing attitude
toward exercise. In 1995, the Centers for Disease Control and
Prevention, the American Heart Association, the American College of
Sports Medicine and the U.S. Surgeon General issued new guidelines. The guidelines emphasize activity instead of intensity because
studies found that less vigorous forms of activity also can improve
your health. *Activity* also became the preferred term over *exercise*
because to many people exercise implies a planned, repetitive
routine. An activity doesn't have to be structured to be beneficial.

Ideally, the duration of your daily physical activity should be
about 30 minutes if it is moderately intense. Lighter activities
require more time for the same benefits. Over the course of the day,
it may be easier to do several lighter activities than to carve a 30-
minute period out of your busy schedule for a structured exercise
routine. Formal exercise is more efficient at burning calories but
requires more planning. Physical activity worked into your day
requires little time commitment if you consider that you can

accumulate your activities in 5- to 10-minute intervals. Three 10-minute periods of moderate physical activity are almost as beneficial to your overall health as one 30-minute session.

Genes vs. lifestyle

If you're still not convinced that your lifestyle — what you eat and how much physical activity you get — influences your weight far more than your genes, consider this. Chinese in the United States have higher rates of many chronic diseases than do Chinese in China.

In an attempt to explain why this is, researchers compared the dietary habits, physical activity levels and body sizes of Chinese adults who live in North America with adults in China. They found that although most of the Chinese adults who live in North America were born in Asia, they had distinctly different lifestyles from the Chinese adults who live in Asia.

The Chinese in Asia consume significantly more calories than do the Chinese in North America, yet they get a much smaller percentage of their calories from fat, weigh less and are leaner. Their diet is predominantly plant-based, and they get about 90 percent of their protein from nonanimal sources. They also spend more time in vigorous activities (for example, cycling for transportation but not exercise) and walking, and less time in sitting than do the Chinese in North America.

Studies have also found that the longer Chinese adults live in North America, the more hours in a day they spend sitting. Chinese in the United States begin to adopt a more typical American diet as time in the country increases. As a result, their rates of many diet- and physical-activity-related chronic diseases — such as heart disease and several cancers — increase.

	Typical American diet	Traditional Chinese diet
Calories (per day)	2000	2600
Fat (% of total calories)	35%	22%
Protein (% of total calories)	18%	9%
Carbohydrate (% of total calories)	48%	65%
Fiber (grams per day)	14	33

(Percentages are rounded, and therefore do not add up to 100.)

Understanding weight control

Have you ever wondered how food gives you energy? Food contains various nutrients — some nutrients provide energy while others help your body use energy. Carbohydrates, protein, fats and alcohol all provide energy. Every day your body requires a certain amount of energy from carbohydrates, protein and fats to function properly. Both the energy provided by food and the energy your body needs to function are measured in calories.

Energy comes in different forms

Carbohydrates, protein and fat found in foods — and alcohol found in some beverages — provide calories. Fat provides more than twice the calories per weight of carbohydrates or protein. That's why reducing fat intake is an effective way to trim calories.

Nutrient	Calories per gram
Carbohydrate	4
Protein	4
Fat	9
Alcohol	7

(A gram is about the weight of a small paper clip.)

Foods high in fat are also high in calories because fat is the most concentrated source of energy. Compared with carbohydrates and protein, which weigh in at 4 calories per gram, fat adds calories fast — a whopping 9 calories per gram. A diet that promotes health and helps you achieve and maintain a healthy weight consists of a combination of carbohydrates, protein, fats and other nutrients and balances your energy intake with your energy expenditure.

Energy balance

Your weight is determined by your energy balance. If you eat more calories than you burn, you gain weight. If you burn more calories than you eat, through physical activity or exercise, for example, you lose weight. If you burn the same amount of calories as you eat, your weight stays the same. Referred to as "energy balance," this is the basic principle of weight control. The number of calories you need each day depends on several factors, including whether you are overweight, underweight or at a healthy weight. Your level of physical activity is also a factor.

It takes about 3,500 excess calories to gain a pound of fat. On the other hand, if your body uses 3,500 calories more than you take in, you lose a pound of fat. Losing weight requires a steady energy deficit. You can create this deficit in two ways — by eating fewer calories or by increasing (through physical activity) the number of calories your body uses. The most effective way to lose weight is to combine both.

A slow, steady approach is safest and much more likely to be permanent. It takes time to break old habits and make new ones. You're much more likely to stick with new eating and physical activity patterns over the long term if you build in changes gradually.

Medical problems

Like genetics, endocrine and metabolic factors contribute to only a small percentage of overweight and obesity. Less than 2 percent of all cases of obesity can be traced to a metabolic disorder such as low thyroid function, Cushing's syndrome or other hormonal imbalances. A low metabolic rate is also rarely a cause of obesity. In fact, obese people have a higher absolute metabolic rate and burn more calories at rest than their lean counterparts of the same height.

Other factors

Sex. Muscle uses more energy than fat does. Because men have more muscle, they burn between 10 percent and 20 percent more calories than women during rest.

Age. As you get older, the amount of muscle in your body tends to decrease and fat accounts for a greater percentage of your weight. This lower muscle mass leads to a decrease in metabolism. Your metabolism also slows naturally with age. Together, these changes reduce calorie needs. If you don't decrease your caloric intake with age, you likely will gain weight.

Cigarette smoking. Smokers tend to gain weight after quitting. A 6- to 8-pound weight gain is not uncommon. This weight gain may be partially due to nicotine's ability to raise your metabolic rate. When smokers stop, they burn fewer calories. Smoking also affects the taste. Former smokers often gain weight because they eat more after they quit. Their food tastes and smells better.

Pregnancy. After each pregnancy, a woman's weight increases an average of 4 to 6 pounds over her pre-pregnancy weight. This weight gain may contribute to the development of overweight and obesity in women.

Medications. Corticosteroids and tricyclic antidepressants, in particular, can lead to weight gain.

Illnesses. Medical problems that lead to decreased activity can set you up for a weight gain.

The good news

Although obesity arises from a combination of factors, the most notable causes are lack of proper diet and physical activity habits. That's good news, because diet and physical activity can be changed. By adopting more healthful eating and activity habits, you can lose weight and improve your overall health. Even modest reductions in weight — 5 percent to 10 percent — have been shown to reduce risks of many illnesses associated with obesity. In Chapter 4, you will learn about these conditions and determine whether your weight is putting your health at risk.

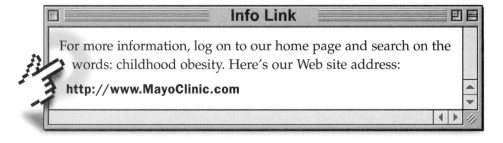

Info Link

For more information, log on to our home page and search on the words: childhood obesity. Here's our Web site address:

http://www.MayoClinic.com

Is your health at risk?

- Obesity is a serious risk to good health.
- Excess abdominal weight is especially risky.
- Even modest weight loss may reduce your health risks.

With 30 billion to 40 billion fat cells, your body has an almost unlimited capacity to store fat. This can have a profound effect on your health. Each fat cell is like a balloon that never pops — capable of expanding and contracting depending on your body's energy balance. When you eat calories that you don't immediately need for energy, your body stores them in these cells as fat. When you eat fewer calories than you need based on your activity level, your body retrieves the stored energy from these cells and uses it.

Excess fat is associated with a number of health risks. Generally, the greater the degree of obesity, the greater the risk of illness. Weight loss can help prevent or reduce the effects of illness. Research shows that even a modest reduction in weight — 5 percent to 10 percent — can improve your health.

Avoidable health problems

Overweight and obese people are more likely to develop a number of health problems. Studies show that your risk of the conditions discussed here increases as your body mass index increases. Your overall risk of death also increases with obesity.

Achieving a healthy weight is not a matter of improving physical attractiveness. Adopting a healthy lifestyle that includes sound dietary and physical activity practices can reduce your risk of serious illness. Improved diet and activity each have their own beneficial effects on decreasing your risk of these health problems even without losing weight. When you combine good nutrition, physical activity and weight loss, you get an additive effect. The three together will greatly reduce your risk of weight-related health problems.

High blood pressure

For both men and women, high blood pressure is the most common overweight- and obesity-related health condition. Obese individuals (BMI of 30 or more) are twice as likely to acquire high blood pressure than their healthy-weight counterparts (BMI of 18.5 to 24.9).

When your body accumulates excess fat, it tends to retain sodium. To dilute this extra sodium circulating around, your body holds on to more water. This increases the volume of your blood. Your blood vessels are elastic but can only stretch so much to accommodate the additional fluid. Eventually, the pressure inside your arteries builds up, and this excessive force makes your heart work harder. Left untreated, high blood pressure can damage many of your body's organs and tissues. Weight loss decreases your blood pressure, which reduces your risk of damage to many vital organs, including your arteries, heart, brain, kidneys and eyes.

Abnormal blood fats

Low HDL cholesterol levels. Studies show that overweight and obesity are associated with low HDL ("good") cholesterol levels. Losing weight can raise your HDL cholesterol level and decrease your risk of heart disease.

High levels of triglycerides. Triglycerides are the form in which most fat exists in food as well as in your body. Your body converts calories it doesn't immediately need to triglycerides and transports them to fat cells for storage. Because weight gain results from eating more calories than you need, it's not surprising that higher levels of triglycerides are found in the blood of people who are overweight and obese. High levels of triglycerides may contribute to coronary artery disease. If you are overweight, achieving a healthy weight will lower your triglyceride level.

Type 2 diabetes mellitus

Type 2 diabetes (previously called noninsulin-dependent or adult-onset diabetes mellitus) is the most common form of diabetes in the United States. Type 2 diabetes reduces your body's ability to control the level of sugar in your blood. It is a principal cause of early death, heart disease, kidney disease, stroke, and blindness. The development of type 2 diabetes is associated with weight gain after age 18 in men and women. In fact, about a quarter of all new cases of diabetes are due to an adult weight gain of 11 pounds or more. The risk of diabetes increases by about 25 percent for each unit of BMI above 22. Losing weight and increasing your physical activity can reduce your risk of this disease. If you already have diabetes, losing weight and becoming more physically active can help lower your blood sugar level.

Coronary artery disease

The risks of both nonfatal and fatal coronary artery disease increase with increasing levels of BMI. Risks are lowest in men and women with a BMI of 22 or lower, but increase with even modest elevations of BMI. Weight gains of 10 to 20 pounds can increase coronary artery disease risk by 25 percent, and weight gains of about 45 or more pounds can increase the risk more than 2.5 times (250 percent).

Stroke

The relation of overweight and obesity to stroke has not been as well studied as the relation to coronary artery disease. But recent studies have shed new light on how best to look at the relationship. Research now shows that overweight and obesity contribute to the risk of ischemic stroke even in the absence of high blood pressure and diabetes (both of which are also risk factors for stroke). Ischemic stroke accounts for 80 percent of all strokes and occurs when the blood supply to part of the brain is cut off.

Gallstones

Gallstones are more common among women than among men. They are more common if you are overweight, regardless of sex. Your risk of gallstones rises as your weight increases. It is not clear how being overweight may result in gallstones.

Weight loss itself, particularly rapid weight loss or loss of a large amount of weight, can also increase your chance of developing gallstones. Slow weight loss — about 1 to 2 pounds a week — is less likely to cause gallstone formation.

Osteoarthritis

Osteoarthritis is a common joint disorder that most often affects the knees, hips and lower back. Excess weight puts extra pressure on these joints and wears away the cartilage that protects them. Losing weight can decrease stress on these joints and improve the symptoms, including pain and decreased movement, associated with osteoarthritis.

Sleep apnea

Sleep apnea is closely associated with being overweight. Apnea means temporary absence of breathing. Obstructive sleep apnea is a serious condition that causes a person to stop breathing for short periods during sleep and to snore heavily. The upper airway is blocked during sleep and results in frequent awakening at night and subsequent drowsiness during the day. Sleep apnea also can cause heart failure. The severity of the sleep apnea is related to the degree of obesity. Most people with sleep apnea have a BMI greater than 30.

In both men and women who snore, a large neck is associated with sleep apnea: In general, men whose neck size is 17 inches or more, and women whose neck measurement is 16 inches or more, are at higher risk of sleep apnea. Sleep apnea is more common in men than in women, and women have to be considerably more obese than men for the condition to develop.

Studies demonstrate that losing as little as 10 percent of your body weight can reduce the severity of sleep apnea by 50 percent.

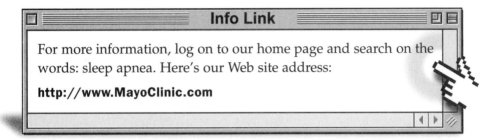

Info Link

For more information, log on to our home page and search on the words: sleep apnea. Here's our Web site address:

http://www.MayoClinic.com

Cancer

Several types of cancer are associated with being overweight. In women, these include cancer of the breast, uterus, colon and gall-bladder. Overweight men have a higher risk of cancer of the colon and the prostate. For some types of cancer, it is not clear whether the increased risk is due to the extra weight or to a high-fat, high-calorie diet.

Can your weight affect your life span?

Obesity does result in earlier death. For adults up to age 75, excess body weight increases the risk of dying of any cause. The risk of death increases faster with increasing BMI in younger people than in older adults.

If you are over 75, you may or may not benefit from losing weight. Talk to your doctor. Depending on your health risks, it may be better to keep your weight where it is. People of any age, however, can benefit from a healthful diet and safe physical activity.

Self-assessment tools

Three do-it-yourself evaluations can help you determine whether you are at a healthy weight or could benefit from losing a few pounds. These assessment tools are your body mass index (BMI), your waist circumference (see pages 16 to 18) and your personal and family medical history.

Apples and pears

Many of the illnesses associated with excess weight are further influenced by how your body fat is distributed. If you carry most of your fat around your waist or upper body, you may be referred to as "apple-shaped." If you carry most of your fat around your hips and thighs or lower body, you may be referred to as "pear-shaped."

Generally, when it comes to your health, it is better to have the shape of a pear than the shape of an apple. If you have an apple shape — a potbelly or spare tire — you carry fat in and around your abdominal organs. Fat in your abdomen increases your risk of high blood pressure, coronary artery disease, diabetes, stroke and certain types of cancer. If you have a pear shape — large hips, thighs and buttocks — your health risks are not as high.

If you have an apple shape, especially with a waist measurement that exceeds 35-40 inches (see page 18) you also have a higher risk of what physicians call "syndrome X." Syndrome X refers to several specific health conditions, including diabetes, high blood pressure, high levels of triglycerides and low levels of HDL

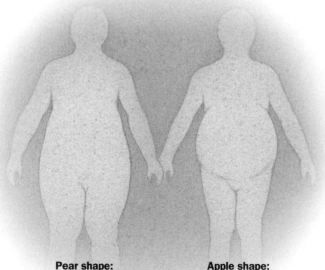

Pear shape: **Apple shape:**
Large buttocks, hips and thighs   **Potbelly, spare tire**

Eating disorders

For some people, eating is not a simple pleasure. Instead, it involves a complex psychologic disorder that may take a number of forms. Eating disorders are abnormal eating habits, including not eating enough, extreme dieting and exercising, bingeing on large quantities of food or purging food, before it can be absorbed by the body, through deliberate use of vomiting or laxatives. Between 5 percent and 20 percent of the estimated 1 million or more Americans with eating disorders will die of associated medical problems.

People with eating disorders often are underweight, but they also can be normal weight or overweight. Women and girls suffer from eating disorders far more often than men and boys. The two main eating disorders are anorexia nervosa and bulimia nervosa.

- **Anorexia nervosa.** People with anorexia nervosa do not eat enough to maintain a healthy weight. They often have a body mass index less than 18 (see page 17). Anorexia can lead to malnutrition, damage to the heart and kidneys, and dangerously abnormal blood electrolyte levels. It also is linked to osteoporosis and menstrual irregularity in women, and a higher risk of early death in both women and men.
- **Bulimia nervosa.** This eating disorder is also known as "bingeing and purging." A person with bulimia nervosa eats large amounts of food in a short time, then uses vomiting, laxatives, or both to purge the food. Periods of bingeing and purging may alternate with periods of extreme dieting. Weight can stay constant but may fluctuate greatly. It can cause dehydration, tooth and gum damage from the acids in vomit, organ damage, internal bleeding from the stress of vomiting, and even death.

If you suspect you or someone you know may have an eating disorder, talk to your physician. Treatment for eating disorders requires psychologic counseling as well as nutritional counseling, and often includes medical attention.

("good") cholesterol. Certain factors have been associated with increasing weight around the middle and syndrome X — smoking, alcohol (especially beer) and lack of physical activity in addition to eating excess calories.

Medical history

Numbers alone don't give you the full picture. An evaluation of your medical history, along with that of your family, is equally important in determining whether your weight is healthy. Consider these questions:

- Do you have a health condition, such as high blood pressure, diabetes or high cholesterol, that would improve if you lost weight?
- Do you have a family history of obesity, coronary artery disease or other illness related to weight, such as type 2 diabetes, high blood pressure or sleep apnea?
- Have you gained considerable weight since high school?
- Do you smoke cigarettes, have more than two alcoholic drinks a day, or live with significant stress? In combination with these behaviors, excess weight can have greater health implications.

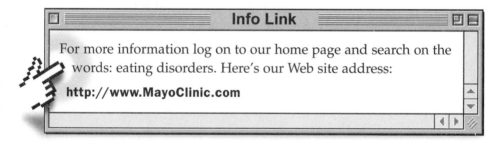

Info Link

For more information log on to our home page and search on the words: eating disorders. Here's our Web site address:

http://www.MayoClinic.com

Do you really need to lose weight?

If your BMI shows that you're not overweight (BMI under 25), if you're not carrying too much weight around your abdomen, and if you answered no to all of the personal and family history questions, there's probably no health advantage to changing your weight. It's probably healthy.

If your BMI is between 25 and 29, your waist circumference

equals or exceeds the healthy guidelines, or you answered yes to at least one of the personal and family history questions, you will benefit from losing a few pounds. Discuss your weight with your doctor during your next checkup.

If your BMI is 30 or more, losing some weight will improve your health and reduce your risk of weight-related illnesses and their complications.

Keep in mind that this assessment is designed to help you make educated decisions about your weight and how it relates to health risks. The information presented here applies to most people, but it cannot take into consideration all personal factors that may affect your weight and health. See your physician or registered dietitian for an individual assessment.

Chapter 5

Measuring the challenge

Take-home messages

- Identify the unique challenges you face before you attempt to lose weight.
- Be sure your timing is right.
- Prepare to make changes.
- Make a commitment.
- Set goals.
- Plan ahead.

It's all in your mind. Of course, we're not talking about your weight. That's as real as the numbers on your bathroom scale. Your fears about losing weight, however, are all in your head. And that has an overriding effect on whether you actually succeed at dropping those pounds.

By now you've heard the weight-loss mantra: Eat less, exercise more. It's a simple concept, but one that's often difficult to put into practice. Every day, you find yourself in all kinds of situations when it's difficult to eat less.

And who's got time for exercise? You can barely get through a normal day, running the kids to school, putting in long hours at your job, dashing to various after-school activities, picking up the dry cleaning, getting dinner together, and tossing in a load of laundry. Exercise? Haven't you done enough?

If you're like many people, you've thought about how you can make it all work. You know you want to lose that extra weight, but you have to find a way that works in your life. Otherwise, you'll soon be slipping back and making excuses. And any weight you drop will jump right back on the minute you give up your new regimen.

If you're reading this book, you also know that virtually hundreds of different fad diets, weight-loss programs and outright scams promise quick and easy weight loss. But the foundation of every successful program for treating overweight remains diet and exercise. You must make permanent changes in your lifestyle and health habits to lose the weight and keep it off.

Identifying your unique challenges

Everyone has his or her own challenges that spell disaster for any weight-loss program. For one person it might be vanilla ice cream with chocolate syrup. For another, it could be salty snacks. Whatever your own weakness, you know instinctively that you should avoid being in the same vicinity with these foods.

But it's not just the types of foods that can get in the way. It can be when, where and how you eat them.

Perhaps you like to eat late at night. Some night owls find they can get a lot done after their family has gone to bed. But if you're raiding the refrigerator a bit too frequently, you must know that it's time to call a halt.

You should avoid late-night dining anyway. Nutritionists recommend eating earlier in the evening so that food will have plenty of time to digest before you go to sleep. Loading up on calories right before bedtime will only intensify your overeating challenges.

Maybe you snack while watching television. There's nothing inherently wrong with this practice, but experts find that you tend to eat thoughtlessly — which translates to eating more — when you're distracted by the tube. If this is your problem, perhaps you should consider keeping baby carrots or another high-fiber, low-calorie alternative on hand, just for this purpose.

Maybe you're a proud member of the clean-plate club. If so, you must confront that urge to eat everything that's set before you. The extra calories don't help you at all, and are better off down the garbage disposal.

Aside from food triggers that will do you wrong, people often sabotage their own weight-loss goals with increasingly creative excuses. Not having enough time, for example, ranks high on the justification lists of many busy professionals. And we've all heard (or used) excuses like "It's too much trouble to cook healthy meals," "I'll never lose weight because it's in my genes," "Ever

Eliminate your food triggers

It's so easy to let eating get out of control. Before you know it, you've downed an entire bag of potato chips or emptied a whole row of cookies. How can you get started on changing those destructive habits? Consider these suggestions:

- Distract yourself from your desire to eat with something positive, such as calling a friend or running an errand.
- Practice saying no to unhealthy food and big portions — and mean it. Just as important, practice saying yes to healthy foods, including fruits and vegetables.
- Before eating anything, picture your action and its consequences.
- Eat when you're physically hungry — not when the clock says it's time to eat.
- Limit appropriate locations for eating, such as your kitchen, dining room, employee cafeteria or local restaurants. Then eat only in those places.
- When you eat, focus on eating. Don't watch TV, read, talk on the phone or work.
- During each meal, keep serving dishes off the table.
- Start with half the amount of food you usually eat, and eat more slowly. Try serving your main course on a salad or dessert plate to make less food seem like more.
- In general, store food out of sight. Put nonperishables in your cupboards and stow perishables in opaque containers in the refrigerator. There's one exception, of course: Keep healthful snacks in a conspicuous spot.
- Don't keep high-calorie unhealthy foods around. If it's out of the house, it's out of the mouth!

since I went on hormones . . . ," "I'm too embarrassed to let anyone see me exercise," and on and on. But what could be more important than spending a little time on your health?

Researchers at the Centers for Disease Control and Prevention discovered that 44 percent of women are trying to lose weight. Almost all of them said they had altered their diet, and two-thirds were physically active. Only 1 in 5, however, was consistent about getting regular exercise and eating right.

Simply admitting your own personal challenges won't get you past them entirely. But it helps in planning how you'll deal with them and whether you're going to succeed in losing weight once and for all.

Preparing to change

Surveys show that most people diet for only a week or two before giving up. If you want to beat the odds, you'll need to think through the long-term lifestyle changes that you must make before actually starting to modify them.

First, you must take a close look at yourself. Consider your

Change agents
How can you get past your own personal challenges and resistance to weight loss? Psychologists describe five stages of change:
- Stop resisting the change. Observe the costs of your current behavior.
- Contemplate change. First, make sure you're ready, then focus on possible solutions, not problems.
- Prepare for change. Set a date to quit your old behaviors, then choose your techniques and tell your friends.
- Take action. Reward even your smallest successes. (But not with food!)
- Maintain the change. Ask key people for ongoing support. Also change the environment: Keep junk food out of the house.

motivation, stress level and your life in general. Ask yourself, "Am I so busy taking care of work and family that it's going to be too difficult for me to commit long-term to this effort?"

Contemplate and write down all the good things about losing weight, such as improving your health, having more energy and looking better. Then consider and write down the negatives, such as adding exercise to an overbooked schedule or getting your family to agree to dietary changes. You can increase your motivation by focusing on the pros and coming up with solutions to the cons. Some experts refer to this thought process as a "decisional balance."

Eradicate the 'D' word

People who are making dietary changes to lose weight commonly label this effort as "going on a diet." But going on a diet means you'll eventually go off the diet, and that can set you up for failure.

You already know you can lose weight initially through a variety of methods, but maintaining the loss requires permanent change in activity levels and nutritional habits. Like any behavioral change, adopting new patterns and leaving behind old ones can be difficult, but not impossible.

Just don't use the "D" word.

Instead, decide on a positive phrase that reflects you and what you're going to accomplish. "I'm changing my eating and exercise habits," "I'm creating the new me," or "I'm working toward healthier habits" might better capture your efforts and the long-term attitude you're choosing.

As you consider taking action to lose weight, realize that willpower alone won't be enough. Quitting a behavior, or adopting a new one, can take anywhere from three to 30 tries. Unfortunately, no magic formula exists for changing habits. Different techniques work for different people. You'll need to discover what satisfies you.

Starting with a commitment

No one can make you lose weight. In fact, increased external pressure — often from people close to you — may only make matters worse. Likewise, trying to lose weight to satisfy someone else rarely works either. You must want to make diet and exercise changes to please yourself.

Of course, this doesn't mean you have to do everything alone. Your doctor, a registered dietitian or another health care professional can help you develop a plan to lose weight. And be certain to ask for support from your spouse, family and friends. These people know you best, and will likely be happy to provide the encouragement you need.

As you're planning to launch your new weight-related lifestyle changes, make sure you've resolved other problems in your life. It takes a lot of energy to change habits, and you want to be sure you're focused on the matter at hand. Timing is crucial. Timing can often mean the difference between success and failure.

When you're thinking about what you expect from these new eating and exercise plans, be realistic. Healthful weight loss comes slow and steady. Try to lose only 1 or 2 pounds a week. And don't keep a picture of a skinny supermodel on your refrigerator and aspire to that kind of impractical ideal. Instead, try to achieve whatever comfortable weight you maintained easily as a young adult.

Make your goals process goals (eating, exercise) as opposed to outcome goals (lose 50 pounds). Changing the process is the key to weight loss. Make sure your process goals are realistic, specific and measurable (I will walk 30 minutes a day 5 days a week).

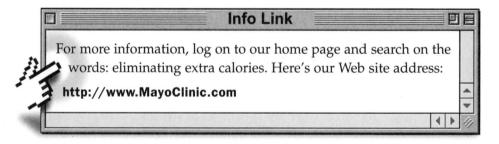

Info Link

For more information, log on to our home page and search on the words: eliminating extra calories. Here's our Web site address:

http://www.MayoClinic.com

Setting goals

Once you've assessed your own food triggers, your eating style, your exercise challenges and your general resistance to weight loss, it's time to work out a strategy that will gradually change the habits and attitudes that may have undermined your past efforts. Then you'll want to break that strategy down into specific and manageable goals.

Choose a definite start date within the next month. Once decided, don't put off that date for anything. Consider how often and how long you will exercise the first month, in 6 months and a year from now. Will you exercise in 30-minute stretches, or will you add activity to your life by taking the stairs, parking a few blocks away or walking on your lunch hour? In general, the best exercise is the one that you will enjoy and do consistently.

Determine a realistic eating plan that factors in plenty of water, fruits and vegetables. Begin thinking of this as a positive experience. You don't want to completely cut out everything you love to eat. With an eating plan that's too restrictive, you'll find yourself first cheating on, then abandoning, your plan.

Write everything down in this planning phase. And go through all the details. When and where will you do it? How will it fit into your schedule? What are the potential roadblocks, and how will you deal with them?

Start small. Remember that you're in this for the long haul. You're making lifestyle changes, and these goals are your first baby steps in that direction. Anything you undertake too intensely or too vigorously will quickly become uncomfortable and you're more likely to give it up.

As you set your goals, it helps to surround yourself with good examples. Magazines such as *Health*, *Shape* and *Walking* include plenty of real-life stories, healthy and easy recipes, exercise tips and interesting facts about fitness. Even if you eat meat, a publication such as *Vegetarian Times* can provide a wealth of low-fat recipes.

Planning ahead

Your old habits may be so ingrained that you practice them without thinking. You can help yourself, however, by raising your awareness of everything you do, then mentally rehearsing your new habits.

Imagine you've been invited to a party where tables will be lavishly set with fine foods. Before leaving the house, you decide how many treats you'll allow yourself at the party. You eat something healthy at home, so you won't be tempted by the party food. Once you're there, instead of heaping your plate and returning for more, you take a small portion of a few items and leave space between them on your plate. You eat slowly and truly savor the flavors. If you're still hungry, head for the fruit and vegetable table.

You can also try envisioning the benefits of exercise in ways that appeal to you. As you're walking laps at the local high school track, think of yourself walking along the high roads of Greece, crossing the finish line of your first 5K walking event, or enjoying the feel of your toned calf muscles.

And accept the fact that you will have setbacks. Instead of giving up entirely, you'll simply start afresh the next day. Remember that you're planning to change your life. It won't happen all at once, but the results will be worth it.

Making the commitment

Losing weight isn't all that hard. In fact, I lost weight many times, but I always gained it back. The problem was that I was constantly looking for that magic pill, something that would work so I didn't have to. Then I decided to take action, mainly because I just couldn't handle the emotional pain of being overweight anymore. At 42, I knew I had to do something.

At first I kept my new plan a secret. Then I realized I needed help, so I told everyone. I even started an e-mail support group with friends across the country, from Washington to Alabama. Just when you're about to give up, you send out an SOS and get back six e-mails filled with the motivation to keep you fighting.

I've had to identify my personal challenges. Ice cream, for example. I know I can't keep it in the house, so I go to McDonald's for a low-fat cone instead. When eating out, I order first so I'm not persuaded by what others choose. I ask for a to-go container with my meal and put half away immediately.

Movie theater popcorn and oversized boxes of candy now yield to pretzels and grapes tucked in a coat pocket. I say no to treats at work until 4:55 so I don't keep returning to the food area for one more bite. I've learned that you have to give in moderately to your cravings, otherwise you're going to eat 20 things and never satisfy your original craving.

Daily exercise is part of the program — and my least favorite — but it's necessary to maintain my weight loss. I keep my tennies under my desk and walk my work breaks for a total of 30 to 60 minutes a day.

I've lost 65 pounds in 14 months and finally gave away my fat clothes. I realized I don't need them as a safety net anymore since I've learned permanent, healthy lifestyle changes.

The night I reached my goal, a gal approached me and said, "You're my role model." I almost cried! I know tough days lie ahead, but I will stay focused and committed, and will never ever give up. The reward of good health is worth all the effort.

Julie
Rochester, Minn.

Chapter 6

Fundamentals of healthy eating

- A positive perspective pays.
- Your food should be tasty, enjoyable and easy to prepare.
- Eat a variety of foods daily.
- Calories do matter when it comes to weight management.
- To limit calories, go easy on portion size and high-sugar and high-fat foods.
- Focus on vegetables and fruits in meal planning.
- Smart shopping is fundamental to healthy cooking.
- Be careful when you eat out.

Adopting a new eating style that promotes a weight that is healthful for you involves lowering your calories. But decreasing calories does not mean decreasing taste, satisfaction or even ease of preparation. You can lower your calorie intake by eating foods that are tasty, healthful and practical. Eating well means enjoying great taste as well as great nutrition. Striving for variety helps you achieve your goals without compromising taste or nutrition.

Eating well — choosing a plant-based diet, which emphasizes vegetables, fruits and whole grains — also will reduce your risks of some of our nation's biggest killers and related conditions. Many cancers, heart disease and high blood pressure, among other conditions, are linked to diet, most notably to diets high in fat and saturated fat. Even without weight loss, adopting a healthier eating style can be beneficial.

Variety is the spice of life

Enjoying a variety of foods helps keep you healthy. No one food provides all the nutrients your body needs. Choose from a variety of vegetables, fruits, grains and lean sources of protein, including legumes, fish, low-fat dairy products and lean meats, to optimize nutrition and taste and promote a healthy weight.

Expand your food repertoire by learning new tastes and trying new foods. Be adventurous and creative! Remember — variety is the spice of life. Try a new food item and preparation method every week. You've probably heard of such foods as mango, kiwi, artichokes, arugula and tofu, but you may not know what they are, how to prepare them or where they fit into your food plan. While you don't need to give up your favorite foods, keep in mind that there's also a whole new exciting world of foods just waiting to be discovered. So go ahead and start exploring.

Expand your palate

Lack of familiarity with a food can easily become a barrier to trying it. Scan the list below for foods that are new to you, then read the accompanying descriptions. Most will be as easy to use and as tasty as foods you already know, if not tastier.

- **Barley.** A grain that looks like rice and is often cooked like rice. Barley is a good, low-fat source of fiber.
- **Bulgur.** A wheat that's steamed, dried and then cracked into particles. Bulgur is cooked like rice. To get the most nutrients, look for whole-wheat varieties.
- **Kale.** A dark green, leafy vegetable with a cabbage like taste. One-half cup of cooked kale is a good source of beta-carotene (vitamin A), vitamin C and calcium. Cook kale the same way you cook spinach — blanch it, steam it or stir-fry.
- **Kasha.** The dried seeds of the buckwheat flower, often ground into particles called groats. Though kasha is not technically a grain or wheat, you'll often find it next to other grains in the grocery store. Like rice and other grains, kasha is usually steamed or cooked in boiling water.
- **Kiwi fruit.** A fruit with bright green flesh and a taste reminis-

cent of strawberries and pineapples. One kiwi fruit has as much vitamin C as an orange, which more than meets your daily needs. Kiwi fruit can be scooped out from its skin or peeled and sliced into salads and desserts.

- **Mango.** A fruit with yellow-orange flesh and a sweet-tart taste. One mango can satisfy your daily needs for vitamin C and is a significant source of beta-carotene (vitamin A) and potassium. Try mango in salsa or fruit salads.

- **Tempeh.** A food made from fermented soybeans and sold frozen or refrigerated in a cakelike form. Tempeh is a staple food in Indonesia. It has a meaty texture and nutty flavor; you can use it as a substitute for meat. Tempeh is a low-fat source of protein, calcium, fiber, isoflavones and natural estrogens.

- **Textured soy protein.** A meat substitute often made from soybeans and spices. Textured soy protein is usually crumbled into dishes as a substitute for ground beef. Unlike ground beef, textured soy protein does not require browning. (You may also find textured vegetable protein, which is used in the same way as textured soy protein.)

- **Tofu.** A curd made from soybeans in a process similar to that used for making cheese. Because it has a bland taste and spongy texture, it's a good flavor chameleon — it absorbs the flavor of the foods with which you cook it. Use it in stir-fry dishes or scramble it like an egg. When it's frozen, you can crumble it into recipes that call for ground meat.

- **Tomatillo.** A fruit that looks like a small, green tomato with a parchmentlike husk. It has a taste reminiscent of lemons, apples and herbs. Tomatillos are low in calories and provide potassium. Add them to guacamole, salsa and casseroles.

Calories do count

In recent years, the fat content of the American diet has been under scrutiny by researchers. The food industry responded by developing reduced-fat versions of countless popular foods. What we have found since the advent of the reduced-fat counterpart is that despite a lower intake of dietary fat, Americans are still getting fatter. The fact is that reduced-fat foods still have calories — some even with as many calories as their full-fat counterparts.

So what it comes down to is this: calories really do count. You learned in Chapter 3 that energy comes in different forms — from fat, carbohydrates and protein in foods and from alcohol in some beverages. Balancing the energy you take in from food and that which you expend through physical activity helps you manage your weight. Because fat has more than twice the calories of carbohydrate and protein ounce for ounce, reducing the fat content of your diet is one important way to cut calories.

Fat in your diet

Zero-fat, fat-free, nonfat, low-fat, reduced-fat, "lite." From soup to nuts, products are labeled with a dizzying array of fat qualifiers — all reminders to keep your fat intake low. But how low should you go? Current government dietary guidelines recommend that healthy Americans get no more than 30 percent of total calories from fat, but this is an upper limit. How low should you go to promote a healthy weight? If a low-fat diet is good, is an even lower-fat diet better? You shouldn't look at fat alone. Fat needs to be considered in the total picture of healthful eating and living.

Fats are essential to the life of all cells. They play a role in your body's immune system; in the synthesis of hormonelike compounds that participate in the regulation of blood pressure, heart rate, blood vessel expansion, blood clotting and the nervous system; and in maintaining the structure and function of the outer covering of your cells. Animal products — meats, dairy products and eggs — are the main sources of fat in the American diet. They also provide most of the saturated fat and all of the cholesterol. Fruits, vegetables and grains are relatively low in fat.

Several different kinds of fat are in your food — including saturated, polyunsaturated, monounsaturated and trans fats. In terms of healthfulness, not all fats are equal. But they all contain the same number of calories per gram — 9, which is why you need to limit all of them in your diet.

Saturated fat

The main dietary culprit in raising blood cholesterol and increasing the risk of coronary artery disease, saturated fat is usually solid or waxy at room temperature. Foods high in saturated fat include red meats and most dairy products, as well as coconut, palm and other tropical oils.

Polyunsaturated fat

This type of fat helps lower your blood cholesterol, but it seems to be susceptible to a chemical process called oxidation, which enables cells in your arteries to absorb fats and cholesterol. It is usually liquid at room temperature and in the refrigerator. Vegetable oils such as safflower, corn, sunflower, soy and cotton-seed oil are high in polyunsaturated fat.

Monounsaturated fat

This type of fat also helps lower blood cholesterol and is more resistant to oxidation. It is liquid at room temperature but may start to solidify in the refrigerator. Olive, canola and nut oils are sources of monounsaturated fat.

Trans fat

Also referred to as partially hydrogenated vegetable oils, this type of fat may be as harmful to your health as saturated fat (maybe worse) by raising blood cholesterol levels along with other effects. The most common sources include hardened vegetable fat, such as margarine or shortening, and products made from them, such as cookies, crackers and certain prepared foods.

Reality check — Low-fat does not necessarily mean low-calorie

Low-fat, reduced-fat and "lite" foods may be low (or at least lower) in fat. But don't be fooled by the fat claim on the label. Some processed foods touted as "low-fat" are also high in calories and offer little nutritional value. Fruits, vegetables and whole grains, on the other hand, are naturally low in fat as well as calories. To avoid the pitfall, pay attention to fat, calories and nutrients in all the foods you eat. All three are important; a mere glance at fat grams doesn't tell you all you need to know.

Also, eat smaller portions of all foods, including low-fat foods.

Handled incorrectly, even a low-fat diet can lead to weight gain. That happens if you cut back on fat but take in excess calories by ignoring the rest of what you eat. Too many calories from any source result in added pounds. Also, severely restricting fat to the point of cutting most or all fatty foods from your diet may deprive you of necessary nutrients found in those foods.

Choosing lean meat

The amount of fat in beef varies with the amount of "marbling"—the white particles of fat that are interspersed throughout the meat. To reduce fat, choose beef with the least marbling:

- Round cuts
- Loin cuts
- Lean or extra-lean ground beef

Also look at the grade of beef:

- "Prime" has the highest amount of fat.
- "Choice" is the next step down.
- "Select" has the lowest amount of fat and fewer calories than choice.
- When possible, prepare dishes with poultry (white meat with the skin and fat trimmed off) or seafood instead of beef.

Carbohydrates in your diet

If you're eating less fat, chances are you're eating more of something else to fill the void. That something is probably carbohydrate. Carbohydrates are the fuel your body needs to function. Your brain, for example, primarily uses carbohydrate as its source of energy. Most of the carbohydrates are plant based. Grains, vegetables, fruits and legumes (such as peas and beans) are typical sources. Dairy products are the only animal-based foods with substantial carbohydrates.

At the base of all carbohydrates are sugar "units." Depending on how many there are and how intricately they're connected, these units determine whether carbohydrates are simple (sugars) or complex (starches and fibers).

Simple carbohydrates are built from single or double sugar units. Simple carbohydrates are found in milk, fruits and some vegetables. However, the main sources in most people's diets are added sugars and processed foods. Table sugar is a pure form of simple carbohydrate.

Complex carbohydrates — starches and fibers — consist of combinations of chains of sugar units. In contrast to simple carbohydrates, your body usually takes more steps to break down starches. Fiber is so complex it's not even digested. Complex carbohydrates can be found in grains or foods made from grains, such as bread, cereal and pasta. Potatoes and some other vegetables, such as corn and butternut squash, are high in starch.

Sugars and starches provide 4 calories per gram, whereas fiber has no calorie value because it's not absorbed. Instead, it helps to move things more easily through your digestive system and can slow the absorption of calories.

The case for high fiber

Health experts are directing more and more attention to the important role certain complex carbohydrates play in diet. Of special interest are foods high in fiber and nutrient rich, such as whole grains, vegetables and legumes (see page 62). High-fiber carbohydrates are digested more slowly and, as a result, your blood sugar level doesn't rise as quickly. By eating more high-fiber foods, people with diabetes can help keep their blood glucose levels lower. By comparison, low-fiber carbohydrates are digested faster, so they raise your blood sugar rapidly. Fiber also protects against heart disease.

How to get your 'carbs'

Nutrition experts generally agree that 55 percent to 60 percent of your total daily calories should come from carbohydrates. Because all carbohydrates are not equal, there's growing evidence that you should be choosy about those you eat.

Steer away from simple carbohydrates such as table sugar and other sweeteners, and limit fruit juice — stick with fresh fruits as much as possible. With complex carbohydrates, avoid loading up on only low-fiber carbs. Instead, try to eat plenty of complex carbohydrates that include a good dose of fiber, such as whole-grain bread and pasta, brown rice, bulgur, and fresh vegetables, raw or cooked lightly.

Setting the record straight — carbohydrates do not make you fat

Carbohydrates don't make you fat; excess calories do. Recently, the popular press has been paying increased attention to low-carbohydrate, high-protein diets — diets that have been around for decades in one form or another but have never been supported by research. They claim you can eat all the meat and cheese you want and still lose weight.

These diets give carbohydrates a bad name by claiming that they contribute to obesity by stimulating insulin secretion, which promotes body fat. While carbohydrates do stimulate insulin secretion immediately after eating them — this is the normal process that allows carbohydrates to be absorbed into cells — people do not gain weight on high-carbohydrate diets unless they are eating excess calories. And excess calories from any source will cause weight gain.

Proponents of high-protein diets insist that eating carbohydrates results in insulin resistance and chronically elevated blood sugar levels. In truth, the causes of chronically elevated blood sugar levels — known as diabetes — are obesity, inactivity and hereditary tendencies.

Furthermore, some low-carbohydrate diets restrict grains, fruits and vegetables, and emphasize milk, meat and fat. Whole milk and meat are loaded with saturated fat and cholesterol, which promote heart disease. In addition, the total fat content in dairy products and meat promotes obesity and certain cancers.

Plant-based foods — such as grains, fruits and vegetables — not only are low in fat and saturated fat (they contain no cholesterol), but also are loaded with essential vitamins, minerals and other disease-fighting nutrients such as fiber, antioxidants and isoflavones. These phytochemicals play a protective role in fighting serious diseases such as cancer, osteoporosis, high blood pressure and heart disease. So don't believe the rumors — many carbohydrate-containing foods are healthful and an important part of a weight-loss plan.

Watch those portion sizes

The importance of portion size is often underestimated. You may think "one sitting equals one serving," but that is usually far from reality. Serving sizes may be smaller than you think. Initially you may find it helpful to measure and weigh your foods. After a while, you'll become skilled at eyeballing the measurements. Using the following suggestions as a guide, you will be able to put away your kitchen scale and start watching your progress on the bathroom scale:

Sizing up your servings	
A single serving of . . .	Is about the size of . . .
Meat (1½ to 2 ounces)	Half a deck of cards
Fish (3 ounces)	A deck of cards
Cheese (1½ ounces)	A pair of dice

It is especially important to watch serving sizes when eating out. Most restaurants serve oversized portions. But you don't need to eat everything on your plate. Use the easy-to-remember tips above to help you sort out serving sizes when you're eating away from home, and save the rest for tomorrow's lunch.

Energy density — feeling full on fewer calories

Feel full on fewer calories — it sounds like one of those gimmicks. But studies show this concept makes sense. Scientists at Pennsylvania State University and the University of Alabama at Birmingham have studied the concept of energy density and put it to the test in their nutrition laboratories on real people. The people in their studies have lost significant amounts of weight and generally have kept a good deal of it off, decreasing their risk of weight-related diseases.

Simply, the energy density of a food refers to the calories in a given amount of food. Foods high in fat often have high energy density — a relatively small amount of food contains a large number of calories. Foods high in water content and fiber, on the other hand, usually have a small number of calories in a large amount of food. These foods are referred to as having low energy density. But not all foods that have high energy density are high in fat. Sugar, for example, is high in energy density. Also, not all foods high in fiber have low energy density.

Picture a 1/4-cup-size measuring cup — it's pretty small. Fill it up with raisins. Now picture a 2-cup-size measuring cup and fill most of it up with grapes. Each has the same amount of fiber and contains about 100 calories, but you get nearly 8 times as much food with the grapes.

You may be wondering how this is when raisins are only dried grapes. But when they're dried they lose most of their water. This water increases the volume of the food without increasing calories. So you get a lot more food for the same calories. Raisins have a much higher energy density than grapes. Strive to include in your diet as many foods that have low energy density as possible. You will learn more about how to do this in Chapter 7.

Food group fundamentals

In Chapter 7 you will learn how to convert your knowledge into action. The fundamentals of healthy eating set forth in the next chapter are based on the concept of energy density and the following food groups: vegetables, fruits, carbohydrates, protein and dairy, fats, and sweets. Here's a close look at these groups.

Vegetables and fruits groups

You can enjoy them raw or cooked, on their own or as accompaniments to other dishes, in soups or salads, as appetizers, entrees or desserts. Vegetables and fruits offer a wonderful array of flavors, textures and colors. They give new meaning to "eating well." They not only provide sensory pleasure, they also promote health through their disease-fighting nutrients. You get a lot for your money with vegetables and fruits because they're high in nutrition yet low in calories.

Most vegetables and fruits are low in energy density because they have a high content of fiber and water — two important nutrients that provide no calories but help you feel full. You can improve your diet without cutting back on the volume of food you eat by eating more vegetables and fruits in place of foods that have more fat and calories. Try a new vegetable or fruit each week. Find your favorites and treat yourself often.

Vegetables. Vegetables contain no cholesterol and are naturally low in fat, sodium and calories. And they are high in dietary fiber and phytochemicals. Fresh vegetables are best, but frozen vegetables are good, too. Most canned vegetables are high in sodium, because sodium is used as a preservative in the canning process. If you use canned vegetables, look for labels that indicate that no salt is added, or be sure to rinse them.

When selecting fresh produce, choose in-season vegetables. Look for bright-colored, blemish-free, and characteristically shaped and sized items. Leaves or greens should be crisp — any sign of wilting indicates it's not that fresh. And buy only enough for a few days. Long storage time diminishes nutrient levels and taste.

Do not wash vegetables before you store them. Put root vegetables such as potatoes, turnips, yams and rutabagas in a cool, dark place and store the other vegetables in the refrigerator. Make sure all produce is dry before storing.

When preparing vegetables, wash them well to remove dirt and pesticide residue. When possible, leave edible peels on vegetables because many contain considerable nutrients, including fiber. If you are cooking them, do it as quickly as possible. Long exposure to higher temperatures leads to loss of some nutrients.

You can (and should) enjoy eating many vegetables raw. Keep bell peppers, broccoli, carrots, cauliflower, celery, cherry or grape tomatoes and other raw vegetables ready to eat in the refrigerator, and reach for them if you have the urge to snack. If you like to dip your raw veggies, make your own dip with low-fat or nonfat yogurt or cottage cheese mixed with various herbs and seasonings, or select a commercial dip that is nonfat or low in fat.

Fruits. Like vegetables, fruits are great sources of fiber, vitamins, minerals and other phytochemicals. They are low in calories and virtually free of fat (except for avocado), so they help you control your weight and reduce your risk of weight-related diseases. Fresh fruit is always best, but frozen fruits with no added sugar and fruits canned in their own juice or water are acceptable alternatives. Use dried fruits, such as raisins and prunes, sparingly because they are a concentrated source of calories, or they have a high energy density — meaning a small volume is high in calories.

Fruits make great snacks. If you get the urge to snack between meals or you have a sweet tooth, keep a bowl of fresh fruit nearby. Fruits are also excellent as part of a well-rounded meal. Add fruit to your morning cereal, to your salad at lunch, or use it as a dessert.

Like vegetables, choose in-season fruits — the closer you are to the source, the fresher the fruit is going to be. Select fruits that feel heavy for their size. Smell them for their characteristic aromas.

Wash all fruits thoroughly under cold running water before cutting or eating whole. As with vegetables, leave on edible peels for additional texture and nutrients, including fiber. Prepare fresh fruits close to serving time to maximize flavor, texture and nutrients. Some salads benefit from a little chilling time before serving for the various flavors to meld.

Carbohydrates group

Earlier in this chapter you learned about carbohydrate as a nutrient (see page 56). In Chapter 7, the term "carbohydrate" is also used to refer to a group of foods — specifically, grains, such as breads, cereals, rice, and pasta, and starchy vegetables, such as corn, potatoes and some squashes. Carbohydrates vary in energy density. Carbohydrates such as croissants, crackers and dessert breads are high in fat and calories and are also high in energy density. But many carbohydrates have low energy density. The more complex the carbohydrate, usually the lower in energy density it is. Remember that fiber and water add volume without adding calories. Therefore, the greater the content of fiber or water, the lower in energy density the carbohydrate will be.

Select whole-grain breads, cereals, rice and pasta over refined products. Whole grains contain the bran and germ, which contribute fiber. Whole grains also are important sources of vitamins and minerals, such as vitamins A, E and B-6, selenium, zinc, copper and iron.

When choosing your grain products, look for the word "whole" (as in "whole-grain" or "whole-wheat") on the packaging and in the ingredients list. Whole-grain products should be among the first ingredients listed.

Protein/Dairy group

Protein is essential to human life — every cell in your body contains it. Your skin, bone, muscle and organ tissues are made up of protein, and it is found in your blood, hormones and enzymes, too. Protein is also a nutrient found in foods. It provides 4 calories per gram — the same as carbohydrate.

Protein is also a food group. Foods rich in protein include legumes, fish, lean meat and low-fat dairy products such as skim or low-fat milk, yogurt and cheese. People generally think of dairy products only as being rich in calcium, but they are also a good source of protein. As you will see when you get to Chapter 7, most of the food you eat will come from the vegetable, fruit and carbohydrate groups. But the protein and dairy group is an important one, too.

Although a good source of protein and calcium (which is essential for bone health), whole-milk dairy products are high in fat, especially saturated fat, and calories. Low-fat (1 percent) and skim milk products, though, give the same nutrition without the added fat and calories. They are relatively low in energy density, too, because they contain a good deal of water.

What are legumes?

The term "legumes" refers to a large family of plants including beans, lentils and peas whose seeds develop inside pods and are usually dried for ease of storage. Legumes are high in fiber and protein.

Some more common beans include black beans, kidney beans, lima beans, navy beans, soybeans and white beans. Examples of peas include black-eyed peas (cowpeas), chickpeas (garbanzo beans) and split peas. Lentils are most often of the brown, orange or pink varieties.

TIPS

- Purchase legumes recently dried — newer produce cooks more quickly.
- Look for legumes of a uniform size — they will cook more evenly.
- Store legumes at room temperature away from light, heat and moisture — they will keep well for up to 1 year.
- Presoak large, dried legumes before cooking — rehydrating them will facilitate more even cooking. Split peas and lentils require no soaking.
- Use canned legumes for convenience — but rinse them well to eliminate the salt that may have been added during processing. Or precook your own dried legumes and freeze for future use (up to 1 year).

Fats group

The fats group contains foods and products that are made up mainly of fats, such as oils, margarine, butter, salad dressings and mayonnaise. Although nuts contain protein, they are placed in this food group because they are high in fat.

An 8-ounce glass of milk contains . . .

	Fat (g)	Saturated fat (g)	Cholesterol (mg)	Protein (g)	Calories
Whole milk (3.5 percent fat)	8	5	34	8	150
Reduced-fat milk (2 percent fat)	5	3	18	8	120
Low-fat milk (1 percent fat)	3	2	10	8	100
Fat-free (skim) milk	0	0	4	8	85

Abbreviations: g, grams; mg, milligrams

The healthier fats include those high in monounsaturated fat, such as olive oil, canola oil and nuts. Limit your use of saturated fats — such as butter, lard and tropical oils (coconut and palm oils) — because they increase your cholesterol levels. All fats, even the healthier ones, should be eaten sparingly because they have high energy density.

Sweets group

You don't have to give up sweets entirely — that isn't realistic. But be smart about your selections and portion sizes. Traditional sweets and desserts are a large source of calories (mostly from sugar, fat or both) and are high in energy density, yet they offer little in terms of nutrition.

Set yourself up for success by not keeping desserts and sweets that are high in calories and fat in your refrigerator and pantry. Getting rid of the temptation before it can cause a problem is both easy and effective. Also plan ahead for upcoming celebrations — a reception, family birthday, special anniversary, retirement party. Cut down on your calories that day, do some extra exercise, or make that event the only time you eat a sweet that week.

The sweets group is composed of calorie-rich but nutrient-poor candies, cakes, cookies, muffins, pies, doughnuts and frozen desserts. These should be limited and, where possible, better dessert choices should be selected — such as angel food cake, vanilla wafers, fig bar cookies, low-fat frozen yogurt, sorbet or sherbet.

Now take your knowledge of the food group basics with you to the grocery store, your kitchen and even to restaurants.

Shrewd shopping

Choosing a diet to promote a healthy weight begins in the grocery store. Because there are so many choices, going to the supermarket can be overwhelming. But fear not! Follow these four simple steps and you'll be on your way to success. Make a list. Don't go on an empty stomach. Shop the perimeter of the store. Read food labels.

Step 1 — Make a list
Using the menus in the next chapter, or using your own based on the Mayo Clinic Healthy Weight Pyramid (see page C2), draw up a plan for your week's meals and use it to make your shopping list. Making a list not only will make your shopping trip more efficient, it will make it more successful! It will help you avoid impulse purchases and cut down on anxiety. Buy only what's on your list. If you generally shop at the same store, keep a master list with items in the order that you travel the store.

Step 2 — Shop after a good meal
It's harder to resist impulse purchases and snack items, which are often high in fat, calories and sodium, when you're hungry. So set yourself up for success and shop after you've eaten a good meal. Sometimes, though, that just isn't possible. The best thing you can do if you find yourself shopping on an empty stomach is to drink some water or buy a piece of fresh fruit to munch on before heading for the grocery store.

Step 3 — Shop the perimeter of the store
Have you ever noticed how the freshest and healthiest foods tend to be around the perimeter of the store? Picture your grocery store in your head and follow the fringes — do you see the produce section, bakery, seafood department, meat counter and dairy case? Chances are you see most or all of these. While there

are some good choices in the middle of the store (such as pastas and grains), most of your selections should come from the store's perimeter.

Step 4 — Master food labels

Since May 1994, packaged goods sold in the United States have carried the Nutrition Facts label. This panel is an at-a-glance method for verifying how a food fits into a typical eating plan.

Each label contains information pertaining to:

Serving size. Look at the serving size and servings per container. See if the serving size is similar to the amount you actually eat. If you eat more, then the number of calories and amount of nutrients you get from that item will be higher.

Total fat. Use this information to add up the amount of fat you eat. For a 1,000-calorie diet, the maximum should be about 30 to 35 grams, and for a 1,400-calorie diet the maximum should be about 45 grams. These amounts will keep fat at the recommended level — less than 30 percent of your daily calories.

Daily values. These values represent the amounts of nutrients desirable in 2,000- and 2,500-calorie diets. The Percent Daily Values tells you how much of the recommended daily amount one serving contains, based on 2,000 calories. Keep in mind that to promote weight loss you'll probably need to eat fewer than 2,000 calories a day. Choose foods that have high daily values for healthful nutrients — fiber, vitamins and minerals.

Some food labels also contain standardized claims. You see them

---

Nutrition Facts

Serving Size 6 Wafers (28 g)
Servings Per Container About 10

Amount Per Serving

Calories 130   Calories from Fat 40

	% Daily Value*
Total Fat 4.5 g	**7%**
Saturated Fat 1 g	**4%**
Polyunsaturated Fat 0 g	
Monounsaturated Fat 1.5 g	
Cholesterol 0 mg	**0%**
Sodium 130 mg	**5%**
Total Carbohydrate 20 g	**7%**
Dietary Fiber 3 g	**13%**
Sugars Less than 1 g	
Protein 3 g	

Vitamin A 4%	•	Vitamin C 0%
Calcium 0%	•	Iron 6%

Phosphorus 10%

* Percent Daily Values are based on a 2,000-calorie diet. Your daily values may be higher or lower depending on your calorie needs:

		Calories:	2,000	2,500
Total Fat	Less than		65 g	80 g
Sat. Fat	Less than		20 g	25 g
Cholesterol	Less than		300 mg	300 mg
Sodium	Less than		2,400 mg	2,400 mg
Total Carbohydrate			300 g	375 g
Dietary Fiber			25 g	30 g

every day — terms and phrases like "low fat" and "good source of fiber." But do you know what they mean? The Food and Drug Administration helped consumers tremendously when it standardized label claims, because it helped to clear up some of the confusion. Check out the chart below. Armed with this additional knowledge, you will be ready to hit the aisles!

Watch for these key words on food labels

FOOD TERM	WHAT IT MEANS
Light	*For fat:* Contains 50 percent less fat than a comparable product *For calories:* Contains 33 percent fewer calories than a comparable product AND contains fewer than 50 percent of calories from fat *For sodium:* Contains at least 50 percent less sodium than a comparable product AND is low in calories and fat
Reduced	*Examples:* reduced sodium, reduced fat Contains at least 25 percent less of a nutrient than a comparable product
Free	*Examples:* fat-free, sugar-free Contains no or "inconsequential" amounts of the nutrient that precedes the claim, such as fat, saturated fat, cholesterol, sodium, sugar or calories
Low	*Examples:* low-fat, low-sodium, low-calorie *For fat:* Contains 3 grams or fewer *For cholesterol:* Contains 20 milligrams or fewer AND no more than 2 grams of saturated fat *For saturated fat:* Contains 1 gram or less *For sodium:* Contains 140 milligrams or fewer *For calories:* Contains 40 calories or fewer
High	*Examples:* high fiber, high in vitamin C Contains at least 20 percent of the recommended daily value for a nutrient (based on a 2,000-calorie diet)
Good source	*Examples:* good source of iron, good source of fiber Contains 10 percent to 19 percent of the recommended daily value for a nutrient (based on a 2,000-calorie diet)

Preparing healthy foods

Healthy cooking does not mean you have to become a gourmet chef or invest in special cookware. Simply use standard cooking methods to prepare foods in healthy ways. One of the most important changes you can make in your cooking is learning to prepare foods with little or no oil. Cooking healthfully is not difficult to do, but it may involve rethinking your approach. Once you get used to these low-fat cooking techniques, they will become second nature.

- Trim all visible fat from meat before cooking and drain off all fat drippings after cooking. Remove fat from soups, stews, sauces and gravies by chilling and skimming it off.
- Use low-fat cooking methods. Choose recipes that call for baking, broiling, roasting, steaming, braising, grilling,

---

Handling food safely

Here are tips for the safe handling of food:

- **Plan ahead.** Thaw meats and other frozen foods in the refrigerator, not on a countertop.
- **When shopping,** don't buy food in cans or jars with dented or bulging lids.
- **Before preparing food**, wash your hands with soap and water. Rinse produce thoroughly or peel off the skin or outer leaves. Wash knives and cutting surfaces frequently, especially after handling raw meat and before preparing other foods to be eaten. Launder dishcloths and kitchen towels frequently.
- **When cooking,** use a meat thermometer. Cook red meat to an internal temperature of 160 F, poultry to 180 F. Cook fish until it flakes easily with a fork. Cook eggs until the yolks are firm and no longer runny.
- **When storing food**, always check expiration dates. Use fresh red meats within 3 to 5 days after purchase or freeze them immediately. Use fresh poultry, fish and ground meat within 1 to 2 days or freeze them immediately. Refrigerate or freeze leftovers within 2 hours of serving.

poaching or stir-frying. Sauté vegetables and meat in wine, water or broth instead of butter.

- Use oil sparingly. Choose olive, peanut and canola oils, which are lowest in saturated fat.
- Use nonstick cookware, which eliminates the need for oil or butter.
- Use vegetable cooking sprays instead of oil or butter.

Finding new ways to enhance flavor

You can enhance familiar foods with herbs, spices and low-fat condiments. Be creative. Poach fish in low-fat broth, wine and fresh

---

Glossary of healthy cooking methods

All of the following cooking methods will add little or no fat to the foods you cook:

Baking. Cooking food covered or uncovered in an oven or oven-type appliance.

Braising. Browning first, then simmering in a covered pan with a little liquid.

Broiling. Cooking food by direct heat in the broiler section of an oven or an oven-type appliance.

Grilling. Cooking food by direct heat over coals.

Poaching. Cooking food in liquids such as broth, vinegar or juice — making sure that the food retains its shape while cooking.

Roasting. Cooking food covered or uncovered in an oven or oven-type appliance; like baking, but usually done at a higher temperature.

Sautéing. Cooking food rapidly with a small amount of oil in a hot pan. For some recipes you can use broths, nonstick cooking spray or water in place of oil.

Steaming. Cooking food in a perforated basket over a small amount of boiling water.

Stir-frying. Cooking by stirring small pieces of food in a hot pan (often a wok) with a small amount of oil.

herbs. Top a broiled chicken breast with fresh salsa. Make meats more flavorful with low-fat marinades or herbs and spices — bay leaf, black pepper, chili powder, dry mustard, garlic, ginger, green pepper, sage, marjoram, onion, oregano and thyme.

Modifying Recipes

Now that you're a shrewd shopper and you've put all the right foods into your pantry, what do you do with them? You certainly can try new recipes such as the ones that appear in the "Color Guide to Healthy Eating" (see pages C7-C16, also 195-200), but you also can learn to modify old favorites to make them more healthful. For example, look at the chart on page 70. Try substituting the items in the left column of the chart with the lower-fat, lower-calorie items in the right column.

Spice up your life!

You'll be amazed at the many clever ways you can enhance the flavor of food without adding fat, salt or sugar. Herbs and spices add bright color, savory taste and sensational aroma. Try a new one every day! Here's a close look at some useful herbs and spices.

Basil. This is an herb with a sweet, clovelike taste. There are several varieties, including sweet basil, small-leaved bush basil, lemon basil and dark opal. Use basil with Italian foods, especially tomatoes, pasta, chicken, fish and shellfish. You can grow basil indoors or outdoors.

Bay leaf. This is a pungent, woodsy herb with a slight cinnamon taste. It is good with bean or meat stews. You can grow bay leaf indoors or outdoors.

Caraway. These seeds have a nutty, licorice flavor. Use caraway with cooked vegetables such as beets, cabbage, carrots, potatoes, turnips and winter squash. You can grow caraway outdoors.

Chervil. This herb has a subtle celery-licorice taste. It is excellent in green salads and good with fish, shellfish, chicken, peas, green beans and tomatoes. You can grow chervil indoors or outdoors.

Chili powder. This is a commercial mix of ground chili peppers, cumin, oregano and other herbs and spices. Use it in bean or meat stews and soups.

Substitution chart

If your recipe calls for	Try substituting
Butter Margarine Shortening Oil	Low-fat vegetable broth for stir-frying. For baking, replace half the butter, shortening or oil with the same amount of applesauce, prune puree or commercial baking substitutes. To avoid dense, soggy or flat baked goods, don't substitute oil for butter or shortening, and don't substitute diet, whipped or tub-style margarine for regular margarine.
Whole milk	1 percent or 2 percent milk
Evaporated milk	Evaporated skim milk
Eggs	Egg substitute. One-half cup generally equals two eggs. You can use two egg whites for each whole egg in most recipes, too.
Sour cream	Nonfat plain yogurt or low-fat sour cream. Nonfat sour cream is not intended for baking.
Cream cheese	Light cream cheese, Neufchatel or low-fat cottage cheese pureed until smooth. Nonfat cream cheese is not intended for baking.
Chocolate	Less chocolate, but of high quality and in smaller pieces for greater dispersal. For a less saturated fat, replace some of the solid chocolate in recipes with fancy cocoa and oil or corn syrup. 1 square unsweetened chocolate = 3 tablespoons cocoa and 1 tablespoon oil; 1 square semisweet chocolate = 3 tablespoons cocoa and 1 tablespoon corn syrup.
Nuts	Fewer nuts in smaller pieces
Top and bottom pie crusts	One crust — you choose which one. You can also make cutouts of crust as a festive pie topper.
Mayonnaise	Low-calorie salad dressing; reduced-calorie, low-fat mayonnaise
Salad dressing	Fat-free or reduced-calorie dressing; flavored vinegars
Ground beef	Lean or extra-lean ground beef, ground chicken, or ground turkey
Bacon	Canadian bacon or lean prosciutto (Italian ham)

Coriander, cilantro. Cilantro is the herb, and its nutty-tasting seeds are called coriander. Use ground seeds for baking. Use cilantro in Mexican, Latin-American and Asian cooking. Add it to rice, beans, fish, shellfish, poultry, vegetables, salsas and salads. Add cilantro at the last minute before serving. You can grow cilantro outdoors. Hang the flowers upside down over paper to gather seeds.

Cumin. This is a small, hot, bitter seed. Use it with curried vegetables, poultry, fish and beans, as well as with yogurt dip. You cannot grow cumin in an average garden.

Dill. The herb as well as the seeds has a light caraway taste. Seeds are excellent with rice and fish dishes. Use fresh dill leaves with seafood, chicken, yogurt, cucumbers, green beans, tomatoes, potatoes and beets. Grow dill outdoors.

Ginger. This versatile spice adds both bite and aroma. Use ground dried ginger in rice and marinades. Use fresh sliced or grated ginger in marinades and with fish, poultry, pork and vegetables. You cannot grow ginger in an average garden.

Hyssop. This is a pungent herb with a minty taste. Use hyssop flowers for garnish and young leaves in both green and fruit salads. You can grow hyssop outdoors.

Mace. This spice is the lacy outer covering of nutmeg and has a mild, sweet, nutty taste. Add it to carrots, broccoli, Brussels sprouts and cauliflower. You cannot grow mace in an average garden.

Marjoram. This herb is a first cousin to oregano. Use it in almost any fish, meat, poultry, egg or vegetable dish, as well as in tomato sauce. You can grow marjoram both indoors and outdoors.

Mint. Peppermint and spearmint are the best known, but there are more than 30 varieties of this refreshing, cool-tasting herb. Lemon, orange and apple mint have distinct fruity tastes. Use mint in Middle Eastern yogurt and grain (tabbouleh) dishes, salads, and with peas, beans, corn and potatoes. You can grow mint indoors and outdoors.

Rosemary. This herb has a piney scent and flavor. It is excellent with poultry and meats, especially grilled. Add it to mushrooms, roasted potatoes, stuffing and ripe melon. Rosemary grows better outdoors but you can grow it indoors, too.

Saffron. This is a fragrant spice that you should use sparingly. Use it with seafood and in paella, risotto, tomato soup and couscous. You cannot grow saffron in an average garden.

Sage. This herb has a musky flavor. It is excellent in poultry stuffing. Use it with chicken, duck, pork, eggplant and bean stews and soups. Sage grows better outdoors, but it will grow indoors, too.

Tarragon. This herb has a mild licorice flavor. It is excellent with chicken, veal, fish, shellfish and eggs, in salad dressings, and with tomatoes, mushrooms and carrots. You can grow tarragon both indoors and outdoors.

Thyme. This herb has tiny leaves and a minty, tealike flavor. Many varieties exist, including lemon, orange, English and French. It is excellent with fish, shellfish, poultry, tomatoes, beans, eggplant, mushrooms, potatoes and summer squash. You can grow thyme both indoors and outdoors.

Eating out

Eating more healthfully needn't confine you to eating at home. You can eat nutritiously away from home, too. Americans eat out more often than ever before, and this is a trend that's not likely to change. So take advantage of the opportunity to enjoy nutritious meals without having to prepare them yourself. These tips will help you eat out healthfully.

Choose your restaurant carefully. Find a restaurant that offers an extensive menu.

Keep hunger under control. Don't skip a meal on the day you are going out. In fact, have a light snack an hour or so before the meal to help curb your appetite and avoid overeating at the restaurant.

Survey the selections. Many restaurants have special listings for healthy eating. Read carefully. The traditional "diet plate," for example, may have more calories and fat than you suspect.

Speak up. When eating out, remember — you're in charge. Ask for:

- Smaller portions
- Substitutions, such as fruit or salad instead of French fries, or skim milk instead of 2 percent milk
- Modified cooking methods — baking or broiling instead of frying, preparing chicken without the skin, or vegetables without butter or margarine. Ask for dishes prepared with half the cheese, oil, sauce or gravy
- Olive oil for your bread instead of butter
- The bread basket to be removed
- Your salad to be served while others are eating appetizers
- Dressings and sauces on the side

Order a la carte. Ordering a la carte can be more expensive, but it's worth it — you get just what you want with the advantage of variety and reduced quantity.

Make a meal from appetizers. Try making a meal out of broth-based (not creamed) soup and several appetizers. Look for items that are broiled, baked or steamed — not deep-fat fried.

Consume condiments carefully. Many of us instinctively add salt, butter, sauces and dressing — sometimes even before tasting the food. Hold back. Well-prepared food needs little enhancement.

Approach buffets with a plan. You may view a buffet as a personal challenge to get more for your money by overflowing your plate. Instead, survey the entire table, decide what you want, and take only that.

Leave food on your plate — or ask for a take-out bag. Eat slowly and only until your hunger is satisfied. If you're tempted to clean your plate, ask your server to remove it. Or ask the waiter to put half the meal in a takeout bag before bringing the food to the table. Order an appetizer instead of an entree, split an entree with your dinner companion, and take any leftovers home. It's easier to control portions at home, but it's also possible in restaurants.

Go easy on alcohol. Those wine lists can be tempting. Whether you're eating out or dining at home, moderation is the key. Although an occasional glass of red wine may have health benefits, alcoholic beverages can raise your blood pressure and triglyceride levels while contributing excess calories but few nutrients. If you do take a drink, count alcohol as either 2 fat servings or as your weekly calorie quota from sweets.

Balance indulgence with moderation. If you're not on a controlled diet, you can sometimes treat yourself to a higher-fat entree. Just balance that choice with lower-fat choices for the rest of your meal. Skip the appetizer or dessert, for example. Or order only water to drink. You also could plan low-calorie meals for the rest of the day.

Part 2

How to lose weight

Chapter 7
Converting
knowledge to action   77

- A new approach to
  healthy weight   77
- Daily dining record   92
- Putting our pyramid
  approach to work for you   94
- Daily menus   94
- Advanced menu planning   102

COLOR SECTION
Color guide
to healthy eating   C1

- Mayo Clinic Healthy
  Weight Pyramid™   C2
- How many daily servings?   C4
- Our best-of-the-best
  food recommendations   C4
- What's a serving?   C5
- Recipe section   C7-C16

Chapter 8
Physical activity   105

- Weighing the merits   106
- Tailoring your
  personal program   107
- The family way   111
- Taking the next step   113
- Crafting a plan   115
- Aerobic exercise   116
- Strength and balance   120
- Flexibility and stretching 121
- Recording your progress   122
- A new attitude   124

Chapter 9
Changing attitudes
and actions   125

- First, think this through 126
- Know thyself   129
- How to change   130
- Deprivation is a no-no   138
- Accentuate the positive   139
- Time is on your side   140
- Put your whole self in   142

Chapter 10
When the going gets tough   145

- Forming good habits   146
- Get real   149
- A solution for
  every problem   151
- Willpower vs. self-control 153
- Friends in need   156
- Staying the course   157
- And finally . . .   160

Chapter 11
Other eating plans   161

- Low-calorie liquid diets   162
- Low-calorie
  solid-food diets   163
- Fad diets   165
- Prepared-food diets   168
- Commercial
  group approaches   169
- Now's the time   172

Converting knowledge to action

- Identify a calorie goal that's right for you.
- Know how many servings you need from each of the 5 key food groups in the Mayo Clinic Healthy Weight Pyramid™.
- Favor the 'best' options in each food group in your daily dining.
- Be aware of the importance of serving sizes.
- Keep a detailed record of your daily eating, and adjust if necessary.
- Eat a variety of foods from the 5 key food groups.
- Commit to a healthy lifestyle.

Armed with the fundamentals of healthy eating, you're now ready to put that knowledge to work. Mayo physicians and dietitians know that effective dietary planning to achieve a healthy weight requires reduced calories. They also know that health, taste and practicality cannot be sacrificed. Otherwise, the plan won't work. Adopting shopping, cooking and eating practices that are acceptable over the long term — meaning they are easy and inexpensive — is vital to your success.

A new approach to healthy weight

Welcome to the new Mayo Clinic Healthy Weight Pyramid (see page C2). We developed this program for achieving a healthy weight based on the research and experience of our physicians and dietitians and the cutting-edge work done by weight-loss experts at the University of Alabama at Birmingham and Pennsylvania State University.

The Mayo Clinic Healthy Weight Pyramid can help you lose weight healthily. Use it as your easy-to-recall guide to the types and amounts of food you need to eat daily from each of 5 key food groups: Vegetables, Fruits, Carbohydrates, Protein/Dairy, and Fats. Our pyramid is based on the concept of energy density and emphasizes lower-calorie foods that help you to feel full.

Research is now showing that satiety — feeling full — may be strongly determined by the volume and weight of food consumed. By choosing foods with low energy density, you can consume fewer calories while still having the same amount of food you are accustomed to eating.

Foods that are high in energy density occupy a small volume, can be eaten quickly and can lead to a large energy intake in a short time. This includes not only most high-fat foods but also foods that are concentrated in calories, such as simple sugars, alcohol, fast foods, soda, candies and processed foods. Fresh vegetables, fruits and whole-grain carbohydrates such as pasta, baked potatoes and brown rice occupy a large volume, take a longer time to eat and lead to a lower overall calorie intake. In other words, when you eat more foods that are low in energy density, it's more difficult to consume large amounts of calories. This promotes weight loss, and you still feel satisfied.

Fiber and water add volume without adding calories, so foods with a high content of either or both of these usually are lower in energy density. For example, which do you think would make you feel fuller — a tablespoon of butter or 3 cups of raw green beans? Even though they contain roughly the same number of calories, the green beans, of course, would make you feel fuller because of their large volume. The green beans contain both fiber and water and, therefore, are low in energy density, whereas the butter, devoid of fiber and water and high in calories, is high in energy density.

Foods that contain fiber and water are mostly found in the Vegetables, Fruits, and Carbohydrates groups. The Mayo Clinic Healthy Weight Pyramid program emphasizes a plant-based diet, and that is represented by both the organization of the pyramid —

Vegetables and Fruits groups at the base with the Carbohydrates group next in emphasis — and the best choices within each food group (see pages 83-88, and C4). For instance, even the Protein/Dairy group contains foods of plant origin and you will find these on the best choices list.

Unique features of the Mayo Clinic Healthy Weight Pyramid
You may be wondering, Why another food pyramid? The United States Department of Agriculture (USDA) has already developed a guide to healthy eating — The USDA Food Guide Pyramid — as a guide to implementing USDA dietary guidelines. While the Mayo Clinic Healthy Weight Pyramid is similar to the USDA pyramid, a closer look will reveal that it is unique in several ways:

- The Mayo Clinic Healthy Weight Pyramid is geared toward losing weight as well as maintaining a healthy weight. The USDA pyramid does not emphasize weight loss.
- The Mayo Clinic Healthy Weight Pyramid emphasizes choices that promote health within each food group.
- Located at the base of the Mayo Clinic Healthy Weight Pyramid, the Fruits and Vegetables groups are the foundation of the program. Mayo's approach incorporates an unlimited allowance of whole vegetables and fruits — a practice first tried by researchers at the University of Alabama at Birmingham and found to be effective for weight management. Vegetables and fruits are low in calories and have substantial health benefits. Most people do not eat enough fruits and vegetables.

What's your calorie goal?
Physicians and dietitians have many ways of estimating how many calories your body needs to function every day. Sometimes they calculate calorie needs by using various mathematical formulas developed through research. Other times they use a machine that measures how many calories your body burns in a day. Theoretically, eating the calculated number of calories each day will allow you to maintain your weight. If your goal is weight loss, subtracting 500 calories a day from this figure should promote losing about a pound a week, because 3,500 calories equals a pound.

In theory, this approach should work. In practice it doesn't. Quite often, people eat more calories than they realize. Therefore, to lose weight, a starting daily calorie goal of 1,200 calories for most women and 1,400 calories for most men generally works best. Over time, individual needs will change based on health risks, the rate of weight loss desired or needed, and individual goals and preferences. Calories can be adjusted to the next higher level if you are too hungry or if you have reached your target weight and want to stop losing.

These numbers are a good starting point for most people — those who begin their weight-loss regimens at or below 250 pounds. If you weigh more than 250 pounds, refer to the chart on this page to learn your starting calorie level. You will find recommendations for achieving each calorie level with foods from the various food groups on page 87.

Fewer than 1,200 calories for women and 1,400 for men is generally not recommended. If your calories are lower, you may not be getting the nutrients you need for good health. Although it may be tempting to starve yourself to lose weight quickly, starving is not a healthful long-term strategy. Besides, you'll probably regain the weight as quickly as you lost it.

Determining your daily starting calorie level

	Weight in pounds	Starting calorie level				
		1,200	1,400	1,600	1,800	2,000
WOMEN						
	250 or fewer	✗				
	251-300		✗			
	301 or more			✗		
MEN						
	250 or fewer		✗			
	251-300			✗		
	301 or more				✗	

If you're a woman and you weigh less than 250 pounds, start at the 1,200 calorie level. If you're a man, start at the 1,400 calorie level. If you are feeling exceptionally hungry despite eating a lot of fruits and vegetables, or you are losing weight too quickly, jump to the next calorie level.

Talk to your physician or registered dietitian before embarking on any weight-loss plan. A weight-loss specialist can help guide you in making the healthiest and safest choices possible based on your individual needs.

Number of servings is important

Now that you know your starting calorie level, you're ready to start planning your days. Below are the number of servings recommended for each of the more common starting calorie levels. These servings will be spread out over the course of your day. If you eat the recommended number of servings daily, you will get the right number of calories. You will not have to count calories, except for sweets.

Daily serving recommendations for various calorie levels

Food group	Starting calorie goals				
	1,200	1,400	1,600	1,800	2,000
Vegetables	4 or more	4 or more	5 or more	5 or more	5 or more
Fruits	3 or more	4 or more	5 or more	5 or more	5 or more
Carbohydrates	4	5	6	7	8
Protein/Dairy	3	4	5	6	7
Fats	3	3	3	4	5

The recommended numbers of servings from the Carbohydrates, Protein/Dairy, and Fats groups are limits, but servings from the Fruits and Vegetables groups are minimums — you should eat at least the recommended number listed for your calorie level. If you're hungry — eat! Starving yourself is not part of this program. Choose from the base of the pyramid and reach for another piece of fruit or more vegetables. This is already factored into the plan. It is possible that the amount of calories you eat each day will be higher than the level you are following, especially since you are allowed unlimited vegetables and fruits and up to 75 calories a day from the Sweets group. So between unlimited vegetables and fruits and your Sweets group servings, you may end up consuming more than your calorie goal. But that's okay. The Mayo Clinic Healthy Weight Pyramid still will enable you to manage your weight while improving your health.

If you are extremely hungry, and eating a lot of vegetables and fruits and drinking enough water isn't helping, you should advance to the next higher calorie level. For example, if you are a woman and your weight is 175 pounds and you're following the 1,200 calorie plan, you should switch to the 1,400 calorie plan; a 260-pound man following the 1,600 calorie plan should switch to 1,800 calories. You should also advance to the next calorie level if you are losing weight too quickly — more than 3 pounds a week after the first couple of weeks. Once you have reached a healthy weight and you want to maintain it, advancing one calorie level should be sufficient.

The Mayo Clinic Healthy Weight Pyramid program is nutritious. It provides all the nutrients you need. The amounts of vegetables and fruits on this program make it high in fiber, vitamins, minerals and other disease-fighting phytochemicals — plant nutrients — while it also is low in fat, saturated fat, cholesterol and sodium. It provides enough protein for proper tissue growth, repair and maintenance, and enough fat to meet your body's essential requirements. Selection of low-fat dairy foods from the Protein/Dairy group helps ensure adequate calcium intake, and choosing spinach and beans will enhance your iron intake. Other sources of calcium include leafy greens, broccoli, beans and oranges. If you're a woman, you might take supplemental calcium or a multivitamin with iron (if you're still menstruating) or both, for insurance.

Food groups

The Mayo Clinic Healthy Weight Pyramid food groups were first described in Chapter 6 (see pages 59-64). Highlighted here are some important aspects of each group as well as best and good food choices, for each group. Foods listed in the Best category are generally more healthful than those in the Good group. The listings are incomplete because of space limitations. Most of the foods in your diet will come from the Vegetables, Fruits, and Carbohydrates groups — all of which contain only plant-based items. The balance of your foods will come from the Protein/Dairy and Fats groups — both of which contain plant-based and animal-based foods.

Vegetables (25 calories in a serving). Most vegetables are included — salad greens, asparagus, green beans, broccoli, cauliflower, zucchini, summer squash, carrots, eggplant, mushrooms, onions, tomatoes and many more. But some vegetables are actually included in the Carbohydrates group. This is because they are starchy, contain more calories than typical vegetables and function more like a carbohydrate in your body. The starchy vegetables include corn, potatoes, sweet potatoes, and winter squash. You will find them in the Best and Good choices lists under the Carbohydrates group (see pages 85-86).

Each vegetable serving is approximately 25 calories. The typical serving sizes are 1 cup raw and 1/2 cup cooked vegetable, but individual vegetables may vary. See the listing below. It is important to note that the recommended number of vegetable servings for all calorie goals (see page 81) is a *minimum*, meaning you should have *at least* that many servings in a day. You can have more if you prefer.

Best vegetables	Serving size
Asparagus	1/2 cup
Broccoli	1 cup
Brussels sprouts	1/2 cup
Carrots	1/2 cup or 1 medium
Cauliflower	1 cup
Celery	1 cup (diced)
Cherry or grape tomatoes	8
Cucumber	1 cup sliced or 1 medium
Eggplant (cooked)	1 cup
Green beans	3/4 cup
Green pepper	1 cup sliced or 1 medium
Kale (cooked)	2/3 cup
Lettuce	2 cups
Mushrooms	1 cup whole
Onions (sliced)	1/2 cup
Spinach	2 cups
Squash (summer)	3/4 cup

Tomatillo	1/2 cup (diced)
Tomato	1 medium
Good vegetables	**Serving size**
Vegetable juice	4 ounces

Fruits (60 calories in a serving). Practically all fruits fit into a healthful diet. But some fruits are better than others. Whole fresh and frozen fruits are best because they are higher in fiber and lower in energy density than canned fruits, fruit juices and dried fruits. Dried fruits are relatively high in energy density because their water content has been removed in the drying process. With the water gone from a fruit, the volume the fruit occupies is much smaller. A quarter-cup of raisins contains the same calories — about 100 — as almost 2 cups of grapes. The grapes are more filling because they occupy a greater volume. Choosing the grapes allows you to consume almost eight times more food than choosing the raisins would allow.

As with Vegetables group servings, the recommended number of Fruits group servings for all calorie goals (see page 81) is a *minimum*, meaning you should have *at least* that many servings in a day. You can have more if you prefer. Remember that your selections should primarily be whole fruits. Each fruit serving is approximately 60 calories. A typical serving is a small or medium-sized piece of fresh fruit or 1/2 cup of sliced fruit. Specific serving sizes are listed below.

Best fruits	**Serving size**
Apple	1 small
Banana	1 small
Blueberries	3/4 cup
Cantaloupe	1 cup
Cherries	1 cup
Grapefruit	1 small
Grapes	1/2 cup
Honeydew melon	1 cup (cubed)
Kiwi	1 large
Mango	1/2 cup (diced)
Mixed fruit	1/2 cup

Orange	1 medium
Peach	1 large
Pear	1 small
Pineapple	1/2 cup
Pear	1 small
Plums	2
Strawberries	11/2 cups whole
Good fruits	**Serving size**
Dates	3
Orange juice	1/2 cup
Prunes	3
Raisins	2 tablespoons

Carbohydrates (70 calories in a serving). This group contains a variety of foods that share a common characteristic — they all are rich in carbohydrates. Some of the more starchy vegetables are found in this group. But most of the foods in this group are either grains or are made from grains, such as cereal, rice, bread and pasta.

The best grains are whole grains because they are higher in fiber. When whole grains are refined, the refining process strips the grain of all of its fiber, several vitamins and minerals, some protein and small amounts of healthful fat. Refined grains are then fortified with some of the vitamins and minerals removed during the refining process, but fiber is not added back. It is best to select brown rice and whole-grain pasta as well as breads that contain whole-wheat or whole-grain flour as their primary ingredient — listed first in the ingredients list — instead of "enriched" or just plain "wheat" flour (which includes white flour).

Each serving of carbohydrate has about 70 calories. A typical serving is 1/2 cup of grain (rice, pasta, barley) or cereal, or 1 slice of bread. Specific serving sizes are listed below.

Best carbohydrates	**Serving size**
Bagel (whole-grain)	1/2
Barley	1/2 cup (cooked)
Bread (whole-grain)	1 slice
Bulgur	1/2 cup (cooked)

Cereal (whole-grain)	1/2 cup
English muffin (whole-grain)	1/2
Kasha (buckwheat groats)	1/2 cup (cooked)
Oatmeal	1/2 cup (cooked)
Pasta (whole-grain)	1/2 cup (cooked)
Pumpkin	11/2 cups
Rutabagas	3/4 cup
Rice (brown)	1/3 cup (cooked)
Shredded wheat	1 biscuit or 1/2 cup spoon-sized
Squash (winter)	1 cup
Sweet potato (baked)	1/2 medium
Turnips (cooked)	1/2 cup
Good carbohydrates	**Serving size**
Corn	1/2 cup
Corn tortillas	1
Popcorn (air-popped)	2 cups
Potato (baked)	1/2 medium
Puffed wheat cereal	11/2 cups
Rye wafers	1

Protein/Dairy (110 calories in a serving). The Protein/Dairy group is a diverse group, containing foods from both plant and animal sources. While foods in the Carbohydrates group contain some protein, the foods in this group will usually provide most of the protein in your diet. Plant-based foods rich in protein include legumes such as beans, peas and lentils (see page 62). Animal-based foods rich in protein include meat, poultry, fish, eggs and dairy products such as milk and cheese. Although many dairy products contain a substantial amount of carbohydrate, dairy is included in this group because it is a rich source of protein.

Because many animal-based protein sources are high in fat and saturated fat, the Mayo Clinic Healthy Weight Pyramid emphasizes plant-based sources of protein. Some excellent animal-based protein sources include fish, shellfish, skinned white-meat poultry, fat-free dairy products, and egg whites or egg substitutes. Specific foods are listed on page 87.

Each protein serving in the Mayo Clinic Healthy Weight Pyramid contains about 110 calories. Serving sizes vary based on the food and can be found below.

Best protein/dairy choices	Serving size
Beans	1/2 cup
Chicken	3 ounces
Cod	3 ounces
Crab	3 ounces
Egg whites	4
Garbanzos or soybeans	1/3 cup
Halibut	3 ounces
Lentils	1/2 cup
Milk (skim or 1 percent)	1 cup
Peas	3/4 cup
Salmon	3 ounces
Tofu	1/2 cup
Tuna (canned in water)	3 ounces
Good protein/dairy choices	**Serving size**
Beef (lean)	11/2 ounces
Pheasant, duck (breast), venison	3 ounces
Cheese (low-fat)	11/2 ounces
Cheese (feta)	1/4 cup
Cottage cheese (low-fat or 1 percent)	2/3 cup
Egg	1 medium
Egg substitute	1/2 cup
Lamb, lean cuts no fat	21/2 ounces
Pork, lean cuts no fat	2 ounces
Shrimp	3 ounces

Fats (45 calories in a serving). Some of the foods in this group may surprise you. In addition to the foods you think of as fats, such as oils, margarine, butter and salad dressing, this group also contains foods such as avocado, nuts, seeds and olives. Whether saturated or unsaturated, all types of fat contain the same amount of calories per gram (see page 53). But not all fats are equal when it comes to health effects. The better fats are those that are primarily monounsaturated, such as olive oil and olives, canola oil, nuts, and avocados.

Each serving of fat from the Fats group contains approximately 45 calories. Generally, a fat serving is equivalent to a teaspoon of oil or a tablespoon of nuts. But serving sizes vary based on the specific food, so refer to the lists below for detailed information. Alcohol may be counted as a fat serving or a sweets serving.

Best fats	Serving size
Almonds	7 whole
Avocado	1/6
Canola oil	1 teaspoon
Olives	9 large
Olive oil	1 teaspoon
Peanut butter	1 1/2 teaspoons
Peanuts	8 whole
Sunflower seeds	1 tablespoon
Walnuts or pecans	4 halves
Good fats	Serving size
Mayonnaise	2 teaspoons

Sweets (calories vary widely). This group consists of sweets, desserts and other foods that don't fit into the main food groups, such as jams and jellies, syrup, hot cocoa, and alcohol. Many of the foods in this group are processed and are not especially healthful. They are high in energy density.

But you don't have to give up desserts and sweets (see page C16). You can eat foods in this group in amounts up to 75 calories a day. You can split the allowance into several occasions or have it at one sitting — whichever you prefer. The key is to limit your intake of foods in this group to 525 or fewer calories a week.

Once you start eating a healthier diet that emphasizes whole foods such as fresh fruits and vegetables and whole-grain products, you may not miss the foods in the Sweets group very much. Take a look at the shift in consumption of whole milk to lower-fat milks. Between 1970 and 1997, Americans cut their whole milk intake by two-thirds, and nearly tripled their intake of lower-fat milks. Most of the time, you can get so accustomed to a substitute food that you prefer it over the original item.

Is eating sugar unhealthy?

Sugar belongs to a nutrient called carbohydrate. There are many forms of carbohydrate. Some have a simple structure; others are more complex. Sugars are generally simple structures, easily digested and absorbed and are ready sources of energy. Sources include table sugar (sucrose), fruits and juices (fructose), and milk and milk products (lactose).

Complex carbohydrates require more digestion. Sources include starchy foods such as bread, potatoes and other vegetables, rice and pasta. Some carbohydrates are not digestible. They add bulk to your diet and are generally known as fiber. Food sources of fiber include whole grains and fruits and vegetables.

The U. S. Department of Agriculture Dietary Guidelines for Americans 2000 offers the following recommendations:

- Limit your intake of beverages and foods that are high in added sugars. These are foods that have simple sugars added during processing — not foods such as fruit and milk which have natural sugar in them. Do not let soft drinks or other sweets crowd out other foods needed for health, such as water, or low-fat milk and milk products — excellent sources of calcium.
- Check the food label before you buy. The Nutrition Facts Label lists the Daily Value for carbohydrate (300 grams based on a 2,000-calorie diet). Ideally, most of this carbohydrate intake should be from foods without added sugars.

The ingredient list tells you what's in the food, including any sugar that has been added. Ingredients are listed in descending order by weight. In addition to seeing sugar listed, these lesser known ingredients also are forms of simple sugar: corn syrup or sweetener, dextrose, high-fructose corn syrup, and maltose. A food is likely to be high in added sugar content if these ingredients appear first or second in the ingredient list.

Keep a food record

Keeping track of the foods you eat is a smart step toward setting yourself up for success. Research shows that people who write down the foods they eat in a log often are more successful at weight loss than those who don't keep track. It's easy and it doesn't cost anything. You can photocopy the form in this book (see page 93), or you can make your own — with a notebook, your daily planner, your computer or whatever else is convenient for you. The secret is to use your food record daily and review it weekly for trends.

A food journal (see page 129) is a record that also includes comments related to behavior and eating. If you keep a food journal, note the time and place you eat, your mood or feelings when you eat, and how hungry you feel before and after each meal.

Keeping yourself on a schedule can help you control how much you eat. If you space your meals at equal intervals, and eat breakfast, lunch and dinner at approximately the same times every day, you're much more likely to prevent snacking and feelings of exteme hunger, which can cause you to eat more than you really need. Regular meals help keep you within your daily calorie goals.

Where you eat can also influence your choices and the amount you eat. Sitting down and eating slowly helps you to feel full, and helps control your intake. With hectic work and family schedules, though, eating on the run is all too common these days. Noting where you ate your meal — whether it was at home in your dining room, in the car, at your desk or in a restaurant — allows you to identify potential problems or barriers to success.

How you feel can also affect what and how much you eat. The key to recording your feelings is to look for trends over time. Some people eat uncontrollably when they feel depressed, while others may hardly eat. You may find that certain feelings correspond with — or trigger — certain eating behaviors. Knowing your triggers helps you to gain better control over your diet (see page 41). A food journal may help.

Sometimes, people eat when the clock tells them they're supposed to eat rather than because they are hungry. Some eat when they are bored. Writing down how hungry you are before you eat will tell you whether you respond to the internal cue of hunger or to external cues such as the clock or the smell of your co-worker's lunch in the microwave. Recording how hungry you feel after your meal is helpful in determining whether your calorie level is appropriate for you. If you feel extremely hungry after most of your meals, despite eating vegetables and whole fruits, you may need to advance to the next calorie level.

The DASH diet

In many ways, the Mayo Clinic Healthy Weight Pyramid program is similar to the Dietary Approaches to Stop Hypertension (DASH) study. DASH was a study completed in 1997 showing that dietary factors can influence blood pressure in a positive way.

The diet used in the DASH study, now called the DASH diet, was rich in fruits, vegetables and low-fat dairy products and low in saturated fat. It was these aspects that contributed to a healthy effect on blood pressure. The sodium content of the diet was moderate. In some cases, the DASH diet lowered blood pressure enough to reduce or eliminate the need for blood pressure medication. These same dietary principles are incorporated into the Mayo Clinic Healthy Weight Pyramid. A more recent study indicates that all Americans — whether they have high blood pressure or not — can lower their blood pressure by cutting their salt intake in half, from 3,000 mg to 1,500 mg daily.

Record keeping is important

The Mayo Clinic Healthy Weight Pyramid can help you select the right kinds and amounts of food. It can also help you keep a detailed record of your daily dining, which will be important for at least the first month.

Use the example below as your guide. The example shows serving goals for a 1,200-calorie diet. Make photocopies of the "Daily dining record" (opposite page). Write your starting calorie level and recommended

Daily dining record

	Foods	Amounts	Servings	Food groups
Breakfast	Oatmeal	½ cup	1	Carbohydrates
	Skim milk	1 cup	1	Protein/Dairy
	Banana	1 small	1½	Fruits
Snack	Orange	1 medium	1	Fruits
Lunch	Greek salad			
	Tomato, cucumber	1, ½	1½	Vegetables
	Green pepper	½	½	Vegetables
	Olive oil	2 tsp	2	Fats
	Bread (whole-grain)	1 slice	1	Carbohydrates
Snack	Walnuts	4 halves	1	Fats
Dinner	Salmon	3 ounces	1	Protein/Dairy
	Salad (lettuce with olive oil)	2 cups, 1 tsp	1, 1	Vegetables/Fats
	Pasta (whole-grain)	½ cup	1	Carbohydrates
	Tomato sauce	⅓ cup	1	Vegetables
	Broccoli	1 cup	1	Vegetables
	Bread (whole-grain)	1 slice	1	Carbohydrates
Snack	Mango (balsamic vinegar)	1	2	Fruits

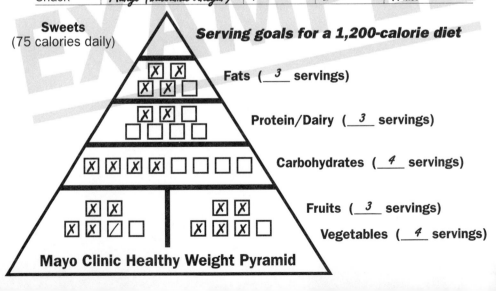

Sweets
(75 calories daily)

Serving goals for a 1,200-calorie diet

Fats (_3_ servings)

Protein/Dairy (_3_ servings)

Carbohydrates (_4_ servings)

Fruits (_3_ servings)

Vegetables (_4_ servings)

Mayo Clinic Healthy Weight Pyramid

serving goals for the day in the blanks to the right of the pyramid. Throughout the day, record what you eat in your personal dining record, including the foods, amounts, servings and food groups. At the end of the day, check the servings boxes inside the pyramid and compare the servings you ate with your serving goals for the day.

Then congratulate yourself, or commit to adjustments tomorrow.

Daily dining record

	Foods	Amounts	Servings	Food groups
Breakfast				
Snack				
Lunch				
Snack				
Dinner				
Snack				

Sweets
(75 calories daily)

Serving goals for my (_____)-calorie diet

Fats (____ servings)

Protein/Dairy (____ servings)

Carbohydrates (____ servings)

Fruits (____ servings)

Vegetables (____ servings)

Mayo Clinic Healthy Weight Pyramid

Putting our pyramid approach to work for you

It's easy to put the Mayo Clinic Healthy Weight Pyramid approach to work in your daily life. Here are the five simple steps:
1. Determine your daily starting calorie level (see page 80).
2. Determine your daily serving recommendations for each food group (see page 81).
3. Become familiar with serving sizes for foods in each of the food groups (see page C5).
4. Maintain a personal "Daily dining record" (see page 93).
5. Focus on variety and good taste. Try new foods using the daily menus and recipes in this book (see pages 95-101, pages C7-C16, and pages 195-200).

Daily menus

For most women, a good starting calorie goal is 1,200 calories; 1,400 for most men. These menus can help you distribute your daily servings among breakfast, lunch and dinner.

Four days of menus are offered at the 1,200-calorie level and three days of menus at the 1,400-calorie level. Recipes for these delicious, nutritious meals are also available (see pages C7-C16 and 195-200). You can move the servings around based on your own preferences, but this is a good place to start.

1,200-calorie meals you'll enjoy

DAY 1   (1,200 calories)

Breakfast	Servings/group
Sunshine juice blend (see page 196)	2 Fruits
2 slices whole-grain toast	2 Carbohydrates
1¹/2 tsp. peanut butter	1 Fats
Herbal tea	---

Lunch	Servings/group
Tuna salad sandwich (3 oz. water-packed tuna,	1 Protein/Dairy
2 tbsp. fat-free mayonnaise, ¹/2 tsp. curry	1 Fats
powder, chopped celery as desired, 2 slices	2 Carbohydrates
whole-grain toast)	¹/2 Vegetables
1 cup baby carrots, jicama, and bell pepper strips	2 Vegetables
1 cup skim milk	1 Protein/Dairy

Dinner	Servings/group
Poached salmon with melon salsa (see page C15)	1¹/2 Protein/Dairy
	1 Fruits
	1 Vegetables
³/4 cup steamed green beans	1 Vegetables
3 cups baby lettuce with splash of balsamic	1 Vegetables
vinegar and toasted pecans (4 halves)	1 Fats
Sparkling water with lemon	---

Food group totals	Actual	Goal
Vegetables	5¹/2	4+
Fruits	3	3+
Carbohydrates	4	4
Protein/Dairy	3¹/2	3
Fats	3	3

DAY 2   (1,200 calories)

Breakfast	Servings/group
1¹/2 cups strawberries	1 Fruits
Omelet with chopped fresh chives (¹/2 cup egg substitute, chopped chives as desired)	1 Protein/Dairy
2 slices whole-grain toast	2 Carbohydrates
1 tsp. soft margarine	1 Fats
Decaffeinated coffee	---

Lunch	Servings/group
Greek salad (Chop into large pieces: 1 tomato, ¹/2 green pepper, ¹/2 cucumber. Toss with: ¹/2 tsp. dried basil, ¹/2 tsp. dried oregano. Drizzle with: 2 tsp. olive oil, 2 tbsp. red wine vinegar)	2 Vegetables 2 Fats
1 medium crusty whole-grain roll	1 Carbohydrates
1 small pear	1 Fruits
Sparkling water with lime	---

Dinner	Servings/group
Provençal chicken and fennel (see page 196)	2 Protein/Dairy 1 Vegetables
¹/2 cup mashed potatoes (seasoned with chicken broth and chives)	1 Carbohydrates
¹/2 cup sauteed spinach with lemon	1 Vegetables
1 cup fresh cherries	1 Fruits
Hot tea	---

Food group totals	Actual	Goal
Vegetables	4	4+
Fruits	3	3+
Carbohydrates	4	4
Protein/Dairy	3	3
Fats	3	3

DAY 3 (1,200 calories)

Breakfast	Servings/group
1 small banana	1 Fruits
1/2 cup bran cereal	1 Carbohydrates
1 cup skim milk	1 Protein/Dairy
Decaffeinated coffee	---

Lunch	Servings/group
Minted Mediterranean fruit mix (see page C7)	1 Fruits
	1 Fats
1 small whole-grain roll	1 Carbohydrates
1 cup raw broccoli and cauliflower florets	1 Vegetables
2 tbsp. fat-free ranch dressing (for dipping)	1 Fats
1 cup fat-free, reduced-calorie, flavored yogurt	1 Protein/Dairy
Iced tea	---

Dinner	Servings/group
Summer savory spinach frittata (see page 197)	1 Protein/Dairy
	3 Vegetables
	1 Carbohydrates
1 medium tomato, sliced, with fresh cilantro	1 Vegetables
1 tsp. extra-virgin olive oil	1 Fats
Sparkling water with lemon	---

Snack	Servings/group
2 cups air-popped popcorn	1 Carbohydrates

Food group totals	Actual	Goal
Vegetables	5	4+
Fruits	2	3+
Carbohydrates	4	4
Protein/Dairy	3	3
Fats	3	3

DAY 4   (1,200 calories)

Breakfast	Servings/group
1/2 cup fresh fruit (pineapple, melon, raspberries)	1 Fruits
1 1/2 tbsp. almonds	1 Fats
1 cup fat-free reduced-calorie yogurt	1 Protein/Dairy
Flavored coffee	---

Lunch	Servings/group
Wild rice-and-chicken salad (see page 198)	2 Carbohydrates
	1 Protein/Dairy
	2 Vegetables
1 small apple	1 Fruits
Sparkling water with lemon	---

Dinner	Servings/group
Thai-style mushroom-and-tofu stir-fry (see page 199)	3 Vegetables
	1 Protein/Dairy
	2 Fats
2/3 cup brown rice	2 Carbohydrates
1 large peach, sliced	1 Fruits
Hot green tea	---

Food group totals	Actual	Goal
Vegetables	5	4+
Fruits	3	3+
Carbohydrates	4	4
Protein/Dairy	3	3
Fats	3	3

1,400-calorie meals you'll enjoy

DAY 1   (1,400 calories)

Breakfast	Servings/group
1/2 cup old-fashioned oatmeal	1 Carbohydrates
Cherries (1 cup)	1 Fruits
1 cup skim milk	1 Protein/Dairy

Lunch	Servings/group
Gingered carrot soup (see page 199)	3 Vegetables
	1 Fats
Crisp rye crackers (1 triple)	1 Carbohydrates
2/3 cup low-fat cottage cheese	1 Protein/Dairy
1/2 cup fresh pineapple	1 Fruits
Herbal tea	---

Dinner	Servings/group
Hearty grain-filled peppers (see page C13)	3 Carbohydrates
	3 Vegetables
3/4 cup steamed summer squash	1 Vegetables
1 tsp. soft margarine	1 Fats
1 cup raspberries	1 Fruits
1 cup skim milk	1 Protein/Dairy

Snack	Servings/group
1 cup fat-free reduced-calorie flavored yogurt	1 Protein/Dairy
1 1/2 tbsp. almonds or 7 whole	1 Fats
1 large peach, sliced	1 Fruits

Food group totals	Actual	Goal
Vegetables	7	4+
Fruits	4	4+
Carbohydrates	5	5
Protein/Dairy	4	4
Fats	3	3

DAY 2   (1,400 calories)

Breakfast	Servings/group
1 bagel	2 Carbohydrates
2 tbsp. fat-free cream cheese	1 Fats
2 plums	1 Fruits
Flavored coffee	---

Lunch	Servings/group
Turkey sandwich (3 ounces turkey, 2 tsp. mayonnaise, lettuce leaf, tomato slices, 2 slices whole-wheat bread)	2 Protein/Dairy 1 Fats 2 Carbohydrates 1/2 Vegetables
1 cup mixed fresh melons (watermelon, cantaloupe, honeydew)	1 Fruits
8 ounces spicy vegetable juice	2 Vegetables

Dinner	Servings/group
3 ounces grilled beef tenderloin, shaved into strips	2 Protein/Dairy
Broccoli in spicy orange sauce (see page C9)	2 Vegetables 1/2 Fruits
1 small baked potato	1 Carbohydrates
3 tbsp. fat-free sour cream	1 Fats
Hot tea	---

Snack	Servings/group
1 small apple	1 Fruits

Food group totals	Actual	Goal
Vegetables	41/2	4+
Fruits	31/2	4+
Carbohydrates	5	5
Protein/Dairy	4	4
Fats	3	3

DAY 3   (1,400 calories)

Breakfast	Servings/group
1/2 cup orange juice	1 Fruits
1 small muffin	1 Carbohydrates
	1 Fats
1 cup whole strawberries	1 Fruits
1 cup fat-free reduced-calorie flavored yogurt	1 Protein/Dairy
Decaffeinated coffee	---

Lunch	Servings/group
Pita bread stuffed with vegetables and	1 Protein/Dairy
feta cheese (1 whole-grain pita, shredded	1 Vegetables
lettuce, chopped tomato, sliced cucumber, 1/4	2 Carbohydrates
cup feta cheese, 2 tbsp. fat-free French dressing)	1 Fats
1 nectarine	1 Fruits
Sparkling water with lemon	---

Dinner	Servings/group
Baked chicken breast with tarragon	1 Protein/Dairy
1/3 cup brown rice with parsley	1 Carbohydrates
Sesame asparagus-and-carrot stir-fry (see page C11)	2 Vegetables
	1/2 Fats
2 cups tossed green salad with 1 tsp. olive oil	1 Vegetables
and red wine vinegar	1 Fats
Hot tea	---
Chocolate pudding pie (see page C16)	1 Protein/Dairy

Snack	Servings/group
Grapes 1/2 cup	1 Fruits
Crisp rye crackers — 1 triple	1 Carbohydrates

Food group totals	Actual	Goal
Vegetables	4	4+
Fruits	4	4+
Carbohydrates	5	5
Protein/Dairy	4	4
Fats	31/2	3

You'll be surprised by these don'ts

- Don't starve yourself. If you're hungry, eat. Select foods from the base of the pyramid — vegetables and fruits.
- Don't let occasional setbacks weaken your commitment to lose weight — expect them.
- Don't try to be perfect.
- Don't be on a timeline. Changing lifelong behaviors doesn't happen overnight.
- Don't give up — you can do it!

Advanced menu planning

Once you feel comfortable with the Healthy Weight Pyramid program, you may want to explore some other options for variety. For flexibility, you may switch off some servings from one group with servings from another. This is another way to tailor the program to your preferences.

If you prefer Asian cuisines, you may want to try a high-carbo-hydrate, low-fat menu, with more rice and less fat and protein. You can increase 2 Carbohydrates servings and decrease 1 Protein/Dairy and 1 Fats serving. Some people prefer a Mediterranean-style, higher healthy fat diet that emphasizes monounsaturated fats such as olive oil, nuts and avocado. In this case you can increase 3 Fats servings and decrease 1 Carbohydrates and 1 Protein/Dairy serving.

When switching servings from one group to another, keep in mind that both the Carbohydrates group and Protein/Dairy group servings should not drop below 3 each.

Calorie goals to keep the weight off

Don't make dietary changes you can't maintain indefinitely. Once you reach your weight-loss goal, you may be able to move up to the next higher calorie level (see page 80). But be careful. Don't drift back into your old eating habits. If you do, the weight will return. Decrease your number of servings if you start to regain weight.

Color guide to healthy eating

Putting the Mayo Clinic Healthy Weight Pyramid to work for you

Variety and moderation are keys to a healthy diet, but a healthy diet alone does not promote proper weight. It's important to eat the correct amounts of the right foods. Regular physical activity is also important.

The new, easy-to-understand Mayo Clinic Healthy Weight Pyramid can help you lose, gain or maintain the weight that's healthiest for you. It emphasizes fruits and vegetables and allows you to eat unlimited amounts of these affordable foods.

The following pages introduce you to this new concept in healthy eating. You'll find useful information on the amount of food you need and recipes to help you get started with a plan that will help you achieve and maintain the weight that's right for you.

Contents

Mayo Clinic Healthy Weight Pyramid C2
How many daily servings? C4
Our best-of-the-best food recommendations C4
What's a serving? C5
Minted Mediterranean fruit mix C7
Broccoli in spicy orange sauce C9
Sesame asparagus-and-carrot stir-fry C11
Hearty grain-filled peppers C13
Poached salmon with melon salsa C15
Chocolate pudding pie C16

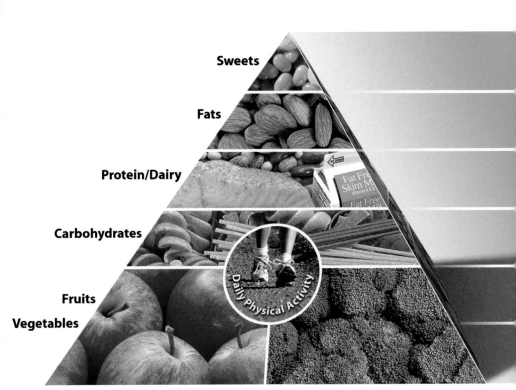

Sweets

Fats

Protein/Dairy

Carbohydrates

Fruits

Vegetables

Daily Physical Activity

Mayo Clinic Healthy Weight Pyramid™

Five steps to healthy eating

Mayo Clinic Healthy Weight Pyramid™ is your guide to the weight that's healthiest for you. Its triangular shape is important. It shows you where to focus when selecting foods that promote healthy weight. You'll also reduce your risk of weight-related diseases. What's more, you'll never be hungry if you follow this approach to daily dining.

The most important foods, vegetables and fruits, form the foundation of our pyramid. But be careful to select from all 5 key food groups in your daily eating. Sweets are OK too, but in moderation. Monitor your daily calorie intake from sweets and record calories in the triangle at the top of your personal "Daily dining record" pyramid (see page 93).

Our pyramid-based approach to healthy weight is simple to master. Think of the fingers on one hand, and then follow these 5 steps:

1. Calories. Identify a daily starting calorie level that's right for you (see page 80). Most women need 1,200 calories. Most men need 1,400.

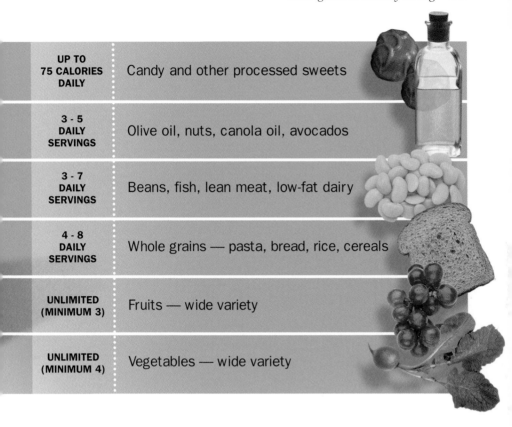

UP TO 75 CALORIES DAILY	Candy and other processed sweets
3 - 5 DAILY SERVINGS	Olive oil, nuts, canola oil, avocados
3 - 7 DAILY SERVINGS	Beans, fish, lean meat, low-fat dairy
4 - 8 DAILY SERVINGS	Whole grains — pasta, bread, rice, cereals
UNLIMITED (MINIMUM 3)	Fruits — wide variety
UNLIMITED (MINIMUM 4)	Vegetables — wide variety

2. Servings. Identify the number of servings you should eat each day from each food group (see page 81).

3. Serving size. Become familiar with serving sizes for a wide variety of foods in the 5 key groups (see page C5).

4. Record keeping. Record your progress. Carefully note what you eat each day, using your personal "Daily dining record" (see page 93). At the end of each day, compare what you've eaten with your serving goals. Then congratulate yourself or commit to making adjustments tomorrow.

5. Variety. The pyramid shows only a few foods because the concept behind the pyramid is what's important. Variety is essential. So are taste and appearance. The menus on pages 95-101 and the recipes on pages C7-C16 and 196-200) were carefully selected by Mayo Clinic dietitians. These foods are not only nutritious — they are tasty, easy to prepare and affordable.

How many daily servings?

	WOMEN (1,200 calories)	MEN (1,400 calories)
Fats	3	3
Protein/Dairy	3	4
Carbohydrates	4	5
Fruits	3 or more	4 or more
Vegetables	4 or more	4 or more

If your weight exceeds 250 pounds, see page 80.

Our best-of-the-best food recommendations

When you shop for groceries, stock up on these foods. Include them in your daily dining. The amounts shown below are single servings:

Vegetables		Fruits	
Broccoli	1 cup	Apple	1 small
Carrots	1/2 cup or 1 medium	Banana	1 small
Cauliflower	1 cup	Blueberries	3/4 cup
Cucumber	1 cup or 1 medium	Grapes	1/2 cup
Green beans	3/4 cup	Grapefruit	1 small
Green pepper	1 cup or 1 medium	Mixed fruit	1/2 cup
Lettuce	2 cups	Orange	1 medium
Mushrooms	1 cup whole	Peach	1 large
Spinach	2 cups	Pear	1 small
Tomato	1 medium	Strawberries	1 1/2 cups whole

What's a serving?

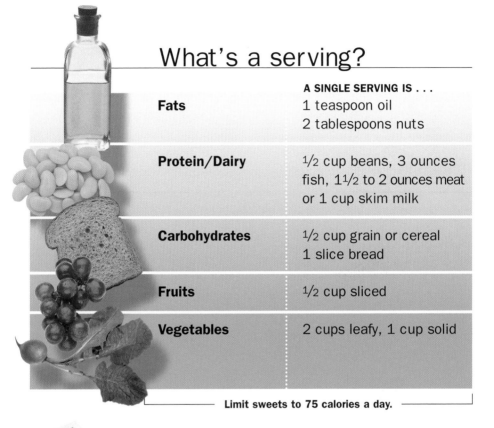

A SINGLE SERVING IS . . .

Fats	1 teaspoon oil 2 tablespoons nuts
Protein/Dairy	1/2 cup beans, 3 ounces fish, 11/2 to 2 ounces meat or 1 cup skim milk
Carbohydrates	1/2 cup grain or cereal 1 slice bread
Fruits	1/2 cup sliced
Vegetables	2 cups leafy, 1 cup solid

Limit sweets to 75 calories a day.

Familiar objects can be helpful reminders of serving size
Deck of cards = 3 ounces fish
Half deck of cards = 11/2 to 2 ounces meat
Pair of dice = 11/2 ounces of cheese

Carbohydrates

Bread (whole-grain)	1 slice
Cereal (whole-grain)	1/2 cup
Oatmeal (cooked)	1/2 cup
Pasta (whole-grain, cooked)	1/2 cup
Rice (brown)	1/3 cup
Squash (winter)	1 cup
Sweet potato	1/3 medium

Protein/Dairy

Beans	1/3 cup
Chicken	3 ounces
Crab	3 ounces
Milk (skim or 1%)	1 cup
Salmon	3 ounces
Tofu	1/2 cup
Tuna (canned in water)	3 ounces

Fats

Almonds	7 whole
Canola oil	1 teaspoon
Olive oil	1 teaspoon
Peanut butter	11/2 teaspoons
Walnuts or pecans	4 halves

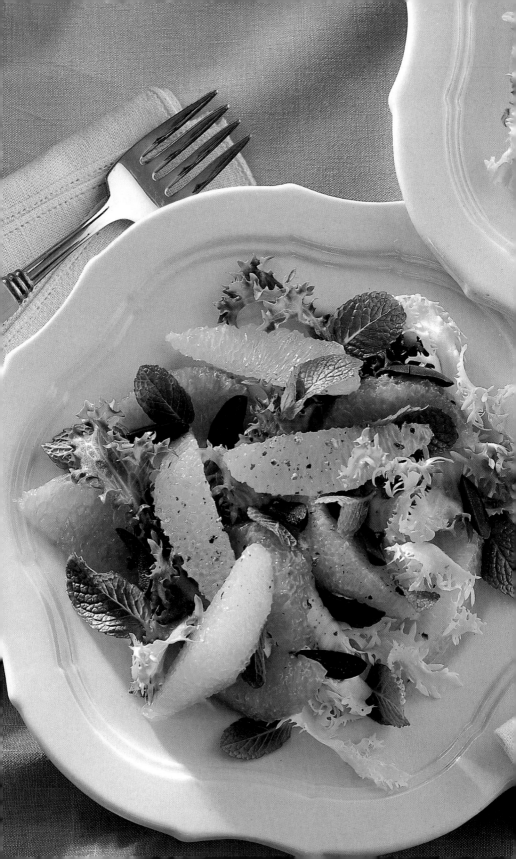

Minted Mediterranean fruit mix

In winter, citrus is at its seasonal peak and is a perfect choice for fruit salads. In addition, citrus is one of your best sources of the antioxidant vitamin C. Fresh mint adds zing to this colorful combination. If you want a nonfat version of this recipe, eliminate the walnut oil and olives.

SERVES: 6   **PREPARATION:** 20 minutes

2 large Ruby Red grapefruits
3 large navel oranges
1 cup (1 oz/30 g) fresh mint leaves
¼ cup (1 oz/30 g) kalamata olives, pitted and sliced
1 tablespoon walnut oil
¼ teaspoon ground pepper
6 curly endive (chicory/witloof) leaves

■ Working over a sieve set in a large bowl, peel and segment the grape-fruits and oranges. Remove and discard any seeds.
■ Pour off all but 2 tablespoons of the juice from the bowl, reserving it for another use. To the 2 tablespoons juice, add the grapefruit and orange segments, mint, olives, oil, and pepper. Toss gently to combine.
■ To serve, arrange the curly endive leaves on individual plates. Top each with an equal amount of the fruit.

SERVINGS IN THIS RECIPE

SWEETS – 0	PROTEIN/DAIRY – 0	FRUITS – 1
FATS – 1	CARBOHYDRATES – 0	VEGETABLES – 1/2

Recipes reprinted from *The Mayo Clinic* I *Williams-Sonoma Cookbook* with permission of Weldon Owen, Inc. The book is available at bookstores, Williams-Sonoma stores and mail order (see page 210 for ordering information).

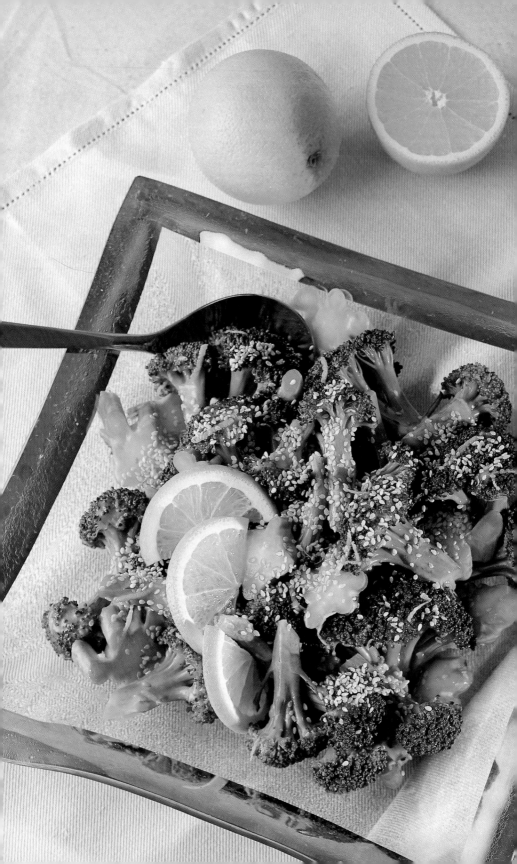

Broccoli in spicy orange sauce

Many recipes call for broccoli florets, ignoring the stems. When properly trimmed and peeled, however, broccoli stems are perfectly edible and supply all the same nutrients as the florets. Some people even prefer the slightly sweeter taste and crunchier texture of the stems.

SERVES: 6   **PREPARATION:** 15 minutes   **COOKING:** 10 minutes

2 lb (1 kg) broccoli
½ cup (4 fl oz/125 mL) orange juice
2 teaspoons honey
1 teaspoon Dijon mustard
1 teaspoon grated orange zest
½ teaspoon reduced-sodium soy sauce
1 garlic clove, crushed with a garlic press
⅛ teaspoon red pepper flakes
1½ teaspoons cornstarch
1 tablespoon water
1 teaspoon sesame seeds, toasted

- Trim the broccoli florets into pieces about 1½ inches (4 cm) long. Cut the stalks crosswise into pieces about ⅓ inch (9 mm) thick.
- In a large pot fitted with a steamer basket, bring 2 inches (5 cm) of water to a boil. Add the stalks, cover, and steam for 2 minutes. Add the florets and steam for 5 minutes longer.
- Meanwhile, in a small saucepan over medium-high heat, bring the orange juice, honey, mustard, orange zest (a piece of the peel), soy sauce, garlic, and pepper flakes to a boil.
- In a small bowl, whisk together the cornstarch and water. Stir into the orange juice mixture and cook until thickened, about 1 minute.
- To serve, in a serving bowl gently toss the broccoli with the sauce to coat. Sprinkle with the sesame seeds.

SERVINGS IN THIS RECIPE

SWEETS – 0	PROTEIN/DAIRY – 0	FRUITS – 1/2
FATS – 0	CARBOHYDRATES – 0	VEGETABLES – 2

Recipes reprinted from *The Mayo Clinic* | *Williams-Sonoma Cookbook* with permission of Weldon Owen, Inc. The book is available at bookstores, Williams-Sonoma stores and mail order (see page 210 for ordering information).

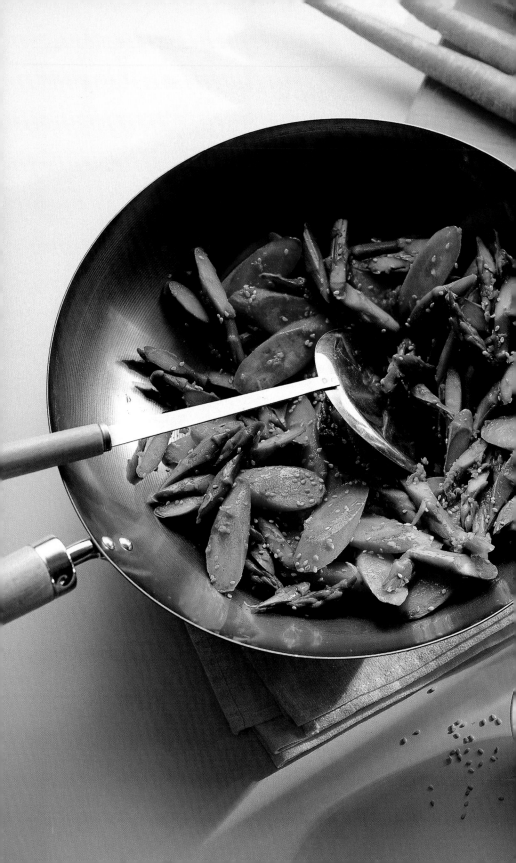

Sesame asparagus-and-carrot stir-fry

The best Asian sesame oil is powerfully reminiscent of toasted sesame seeds and neither harsh nor bitter. Buy it in small bottles and keep trying new ones until you find the brand you like best. Remember, it takes just a small amount of sesame oil to impart its nutty flavor.

SERVES: 6   **PREPARATION:** 15 minutes   **COOKING:** 10 minutes

24 asparagus stalks
6 large carrots
¼ cup (2 fl oz/60 mL) water
1 tablespoon grated fresh ginger
1 tablespoon reduced-sodium soy sauce
1½ teaspoons sesame oil
1 tablespoon sesame seeds, toasted

- Cut the asparagus into ½-inch-thick (12 mm) slices. Cut the carrots into ¼-inch-thick (6 mm) slices.
- Coat a nonstick wok or a large frying pan with nonstick cooking spray and place over high heat. Add the carrots and stir-fry for 4 minutes. Add the asparagus and water, and stir and toss to combine. Cover and cook until the vegetables are barely tender, about 2 minutes.
- Uncover and add the ginger. Stir-fry until any remaining water evaporates, 1–2 minutes.
- Add the soy sauce, sesame oil, and sesame seeds. Stir-fry to coat the vegetables evenly.
- To serve, divide among individual plates.

SERVINGS IN THIS RECIPE

SWEETS – 0	PROTEIN/DAIRY – 0	FRUITS – 0
FATS – 1/2	CARBOHYDRATES – 0	VEGETABLES – 2

Recipes reprinted from *The Mayo Clinic I Williams-Sonoma Cookbook* with permission of Weldon Owen, Inc. The book is available at bookstores, Williams-Sonoma stores and mail order (see page 210 for ordering information).

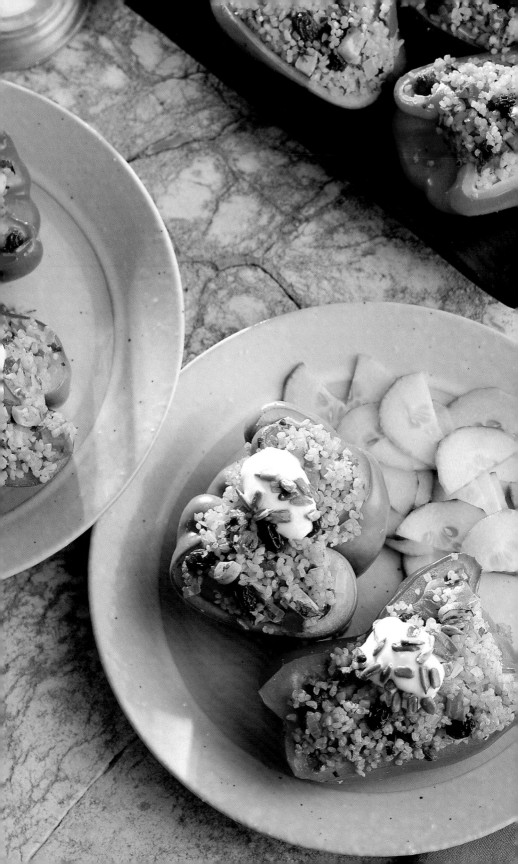

Hearty grain-filled peppers

Enjoy the homey goodness of meatless stuffed bell peppers, which are filled in this recipe with a robust low-fat combination of cracked wheat, mushrooms, tomatoes, onions, and garlic. Complement them with a refreshing vegetable.

SERVES: 6　　**PREPARATION:** 25 minutes　　**COOKING:** 1 hour

4 cups (32 fl oz/1 liter) water
1/2 teaspoon ground cinnamon
1/2 teaspoon ground cumin
2 cups (12 oz/375 g) bulgur wheat
8 oz (250 g) white mushrooms, coarsely chopped
1 1/2 cups (9 oz/280 g) diced fresh tomatoes or 14 1/2 oz (455 g) canned diced tomatoes, drained
1 onion, finely chopped
2 garlic cloves, minced
1/2 cup (1/2 oz/15 g) chopped fresh flat-leaf (Italian) parsley
1/3 cup (2 oz/60 g) raisins
3 red bell peppers halved, stemmed, and seeded
3 green bell peppers halved, stemmed, and seeded
6 tablespoons (3 oz/90 g) plain nonfat yogurt
1 tablespoon sunflower seeds, toasted

■ In a large saucepan, bring the water, cinnamon, and cumin to a boil. Stir in the bulgur. When the water returns to a boil, reduce heat to low. Cover and simmer until the water is absorbed, about 15 minutes.
■ In a large frying pan over medium heat, combine the mushrooms, tomatoes, onion, garlic, and parsley. Cover and cook, stirring occasionally, until the vegetables are tender but not mushy, about 10 minutes.
■ Stir the mushroom mixture and raisins into the cooked bulgur.
■ Preheat an oven to 400 F (200 C). Coat a shallow baking dish with non-stick cooking spray.
■ Arrange the bell pepper halves in a single layer, cut side up, in the prepared pan. Divide the bulgur mixture equally among the bell peppers, mounding slightly. Cover tightly with aluminum foil and bake until the peppers are tender and the filling is heated through, about 45 minutes.
■ To serve, place 2 bell pepper halves on individual plates. Top each with 1/2 tablespoon of the yogurt. Garnish with the sunflower seeds.

SERVINGS IN THIS RECIPE

SWEETS – 0	PROTEIN/DAIRY – 0	FRUITS – 0
FATS – 0	CARBOHYDRATES – 3	VEGETABLES – 3

Recipes reprinted from *The Mayo Clinic* | *Williams-Sonoma Cookbook* with permission of Weldon Owen, Inc. The book is available at bookstores, Williams-Sonoma stores and mail order (see page 210 for ordering information).

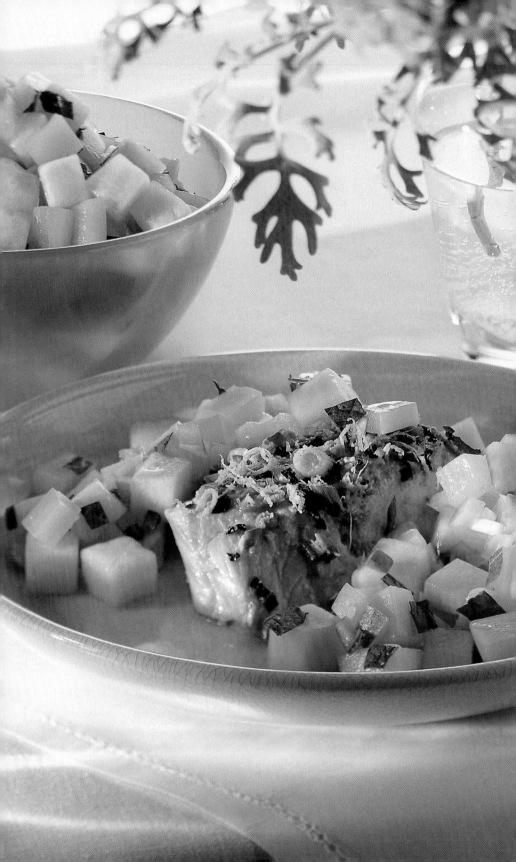

Poached salmon with melon salsa

Oven-poaching seafood inside a foil envelope, a technique called en papillote *in French, seals in moisture and flavor and greets diners with a burst of fragrant steam when the packets are carefully opened. In a practice common in tropical kitchens, fresh fruit tops the fish.*

SERVES: 6   **PREPARATION:** 40 minutes   **COOKING:** 15 minutes

2 green (spring) onions, thinly sliced, including green portions
1¹/₂ teaspoons chopped fresh mint
1 teaspoon grated fresh ginger
3 tablespoons grated lime zest
1¹/₂ lb (750 g) salmon fillets, skinned and cut into 6 pieces

Melon Salsa
1 honeydew melon, about 3 lb (1.5 kg), peeled, seeded, and cut into ¹/₂-inch (12 mm) cubes
1 yellow bell pepper seeded, stemmed, and cut into ¹/₂-inch (12 mm) squares
¹/₄ cup (2 fl oz/60 mL) lime juice
¹/₂ red or Spanish onion, chopped
1 jalapeño chili, minced
2 tablespoons chopped fresh mint

- Preheat an oven to 450 F (230 C).
- In a small bowl, toss together the onions, mint, ginger, and lime zest (peel).
- Place 6 pieces of aluminum foil, each 10 inches (25 cm) square, on a work surface. Place a piece of salmon in the center of each square. Top each with an equal amount of the onion mixture. Fold in the edges of the foil and crimp to seal. Place the packets in a single layer on a baking sheet and bake until opaque throughout, 12–15 minutes.
- Meanwhile, to make the salsa, in a medium bowl, toss together the melon, pepper, lime juice, onion, jalapeño, and mint.
- To serve, transfer the contents of each packet onto an individual plate. Top each with an equal amount of the salsa.

SERVINGS IN THIS RECIPE

SWEETS – 0	PROTEIN/DAIRY – 1 1/2	FRUITS – 1
FATS – 0	CARBOHYDRATES – 0	VEGETABLES – 1

Recipes reprinted from *The Mayo Clinic | Williams-Sonoma Cookbook* with permission of Weldon Owen, Inc. The book is available at bookstores, Williams-Sonoma stores and mail order (see page 210 for ordering information).

Chocolate pudding pie

SERVES: 8   **PREPARATION:** 30 minutes   **COOKING:** 30 minutes   **CHILLING:** 2 hours

Crust	*Filling*
8 whole graham crackers (whole-meal biscuits)	1/3 cup (1½ oz/45 g) cornstarch (cornflour)
2/3 cup (2 oz/60 g) 100% unprocessed wheat bran	1/3 cup (5 oz/155 g) sugar
2 tablespoons sugar	1/3 cup (1 oz/30 g) unsweetened cocoa powder
1/4 teaspoon ground cinnamon	3½ cups (28 fl oz/875 mL) nonfat milk
2 egg whites	2 teaspoons vanilla extract (essence)
	16 strawberries, hulled

- Preheat an oven to 350 F (180 C). Coat a 9-inch (23 cm) pie pan with nonstick cooking spray.
- To make the crust, in a food processor, process the graham crackers and wheat bran to fine crumbs. Add the sugar, cinnamon, and egg whites and process just until all the crumbs are dampened.
- Put the mixture in the prepared pan and firmly pat and press it over the bottom and sides of the pan, taking care not to make the edges too thick.
- Bake until the crust has browned lightly, feels firm but not hard and gives to moderate pressure, about 15 minutes. If overbaked, it will be brittle when cold. Cool completely, about 1 hour.
- To make the filling, into a heavy saucepan, sift together the cornstarch, sugar, and cocoa powder. Gradually whisk in the milk. Place over medium heat and cook, whisking almost constantly, until the mixture thickens and boils, about 7 minutes. Reduce heat to medium-low and boil gently, whisking constantly, 2 minutes longer. Remove from heat and press a piece of plastic wrap directly onto the surface of the mixture to prevent a skin from forming. Cool for 30 minutes.
- Remove the plastic wrap from the filling and stir in the vanilla. Pour the filling into the crust and refrigerate until set, at least 2 hours.
- To serve, cut into wedges. Garnish with the berries.

SERVINGS IN THIS RECIPE

SWEETS – 50 calories
FATS – 0
PROTEIN/DAIRY – 1
CARBOHYDRATES – 1/2
FRUITS – 1/2
VEGETABLES – 0

Recipes reprinted from *The Mayo Clinic | Williams-Sonoma Cookbook* with permission of Weldon Owen, Inc. The book is available at bookstores, Williams-Sonoma stores and mail order (see page 210 for ordering information).

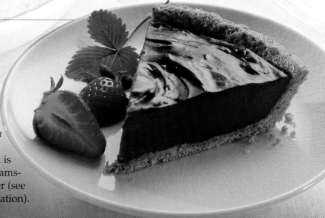

There is no 'Mayo Clinic Diet'

It seems to be seasonal. Usually in the spring, Mayo Clinic gets deluged with phone calls inquiring about the so-called Mayo Clinic Diet, various versions of which have sprouted up across the country and around the world for decades. The problem and the truth: There is no Mayo Clinic Diet.

No one knows the origin of the diet myth, but Mayo dietitians say that it has been around since the 1940s. Over the years, the supposed Mayo Clinic Diet has emerged in many forms, but all share a common characteristic: They are "one-size-fits-all" diets. They also limit variety of foods and promise dramatic weight loss. These are sure signs of a hoax.

A diet is likely to be a fad if it is not tailored specifically for you and your individual needs. Mayo Clinic tailors weight-loss plans to the individual. Each plan includes what and how much to eat, exercise tips and other health-promoting habits.

So the next time you hear about the so-called Mayo Clinic Diet, help dispel the myth by sharing your knowledge.

Your new way of eating

If you take the approach to eating symbolized by the Mayo Clinic Healthy Weight Pyramid, you'll get a balanced diet, you'll never be hungry and you'll be well positioned to achieve the weight that's best for you. If you implement your activity recommendations as well, you'll lose weight, if you need to, and the pounds will stay off.

Your health will improve as the diet and activity changes you commit to become a comfortable part of your lifestyle. This approach works. It is more realistic than following a diet and losing weight for a short period, only to have the weight return when you go off your diet.

Although our program may not yield the purportedly successful results of some of the popular quick-weight-loss plans, it offers a permanent solution to the problem of overweight or obesity.

Passing the test

Mayo Clinic on Healthy Weight and the new Mayo Clinic Healthy Weight Pyramid stack up well next to federal nutrition recommendations. Below, the latest edition of the USDA's Dietary Guidelines for Americans is compared with Mayo's approach. A check in the Mayo column indicates consistency.

Dietary Guidelines for Americans	Mayo approach
1. Aim for a healthy weight.	✓
2. Be physically active every day.	✓
3. Let the Food Guide Pyramid guide your food choices.	Incorporates Mayo Clinic Pyramid
4. Choose a variety of grains daily, especially whole grains.	✓
5. Choose a variety of fruits and vegetables daily.	✓
6. Keep food safe to eat.	✓
7. Choose a diet that is low in saturated fat and cholesterol and moderate in total fat.	✓
8. Choose beverages and foods that limit your intake of sugars.	✓
9. Choose and prepare foods with less salt.	✓
10. If you drink alcoholic beverages, do so in moderation.	✓

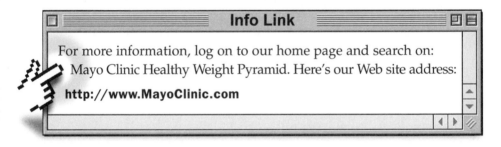

Info Link

For more information, log on to our home page and search on: Mayo Clinic Healthy Weight Pyramid. Here's our Web site address:

http://www.MayoClinic.com

Physical activity

- Any physical activity is good activity.
- Physical *activity* and physical *exercise* are two different things.
- Activity of all kinds burns calories.
- Even with physical limitations, some activities can be performed.
- Physical activity will improve your health as well as your weight.

Match the healthy eating habits from previous chapters with what you find here and you'll have a winning combination that results in improved health, better weight management, and all-around physical fitness.

It's human nature to seek a quick fix, a diet that will take off the pounds easily and safely with minimal effort. But studies show that people who want to optimize their weight loss — and those who stand the best chance of keeping the pounds off — must do more than transform their eating habits. They must make physical activity and physical exercise (two different things) a part of their plan.

Does this mean you have to squeeze into a Spandex suit, join a health club or spend hours every day seeking that endorphin high? It does not. Physical *exercise* is a more structured, planned approach. Physical *activity* occurs from the moment you slip out of bed in the morning until you get back in. Almost every motion of your body is beneficial. Physical activities, such as mowing the lawn or taking the stairs instead of the elevator, are healthful as well, and important to weight management.

You can increase your cardiovascular fitness level with as few as 30 minutes of low to moderately intense physical activity a day. And you can select activities you enjoy. In fact, the smartest thing you will ever do for your body is to find one or more physical activities you really enjoy and do them on a regular basis. When you're engaged in exercise you enjoy, you're much more likely to keep at it and reap the rewards.

Of course you're busy. In our increasingly hectic society, many people believe that even a half-hour a day is too much to ask. But it really isn't that hard. In fact, 30 minutes a day need not be done at one time. You can break up the 30 minutes into two 15-minute sessions, or three 10-minute intervals, and still reap the benefits.

Even though you live and work in this fast-paced, automated world, make the decision to carve out 30 minutes from your day as an investment in yourself, your family and your future. You'll lose weight, if that's your goal. But you'll also live a richer, healthier, happier life. And that will deliver an enormous pay-off for a modest time invested.

Weighing the merits

Adding physical activity to your life doesn't mean wearing a sweatsuit every day. Simple modifications in your lifestyle will help. It's human nature to use step-saving activities. But to improve health and manage weight you should be doing just the opposite: looking for excuses to get more activity into your daily life.

A few minutes of walking or stair climbing can be as good for you as structured exercise. In fact, several studies have shown that moderate-intensity lifestyle activities can lower blood cholesterol, blood pressure, and percentage of body fat, and can improve cardiovascular fitness as well as structured exercise programs.

Should you abandon structured exercise and switch to lifestyle activities alone? Not at all. Structured exercise in longer sessions is more efficient at burning calories. But any activity is good activity. Lifestyle activity is a good start to give you some of the same calorie-burning benefits of exercise. Also, it can be easier to fit into your day. Simply incorporate more physical activity into the things you already do. Stair climbing, walking, gardening, mowing — all of these make you healthier.

Think, for example, about how you could increase your walking activity by parking farther away from your ultimate destination, taking a walk at lunchtime, or adding a few laps to your trip to the mall.

Are you a fidgeter?

When it comes to lifestyle activity, some people have a built-in mechanism for keeping weight off through their own everyday movements. A recent Mayo Clinic study suggests that people who fidget burn hundreds of extra calories. Fidgeting appears to help them control their weight even when they overeat.

In the study, the people who gained the least weight were those who had the biggest increase in calories burned during the normal activities of daily living, such as fidgeting, moving around and changing posture. The researchers labeled this factor NEAT (for nonexercise activity thermogenesis).

The study provides an optimistic message, even if you're not a fidgeter: Every calorie you burn by moving around counts. That means there's a range of extra calories you can burn every day. If you increase that range a little bit, you'll tend to stay leaner than if you just sit still too much.

Tailoring your personal program

No matter what kind of exercise you choose, remember that it's important to tailor the activity to your ability. If you have a chronic condition, a physical disability or other health consideration, you'll want to devise a routine that gives you the optimal benefits with the least chance of discomfort or injury. Your doctor can help you design a program that's right for you.

At one time, many physical conditions curtailed activity in those who had them. But now, doctors recommend some sort of exercise for all kinds of formerly sedentary people, those with everything

Living the active life

Although you'll gain greater health benefits with higher-intensity exercise that lasts 30 minutes or more, low- to moderate-intensity activities can complement your physical routine. Instead of building your life around exercise, build exercise around your life. Here are simple ways to get more physical, no matter what your particular role in life is. Try to add a new or different activity each week:

STAY-AT-HOME PARENT
- Sweep floors, patio and front walk every day.
- Play with your kids instead of watching them play. Go to the park. Push your children in a stroller. Play ball.
- Go for a short walk before breakfast, lunch or dinner.
- Bike to the store.
- Park at the opposite end of the mall from your destination. While shopping, walk around the mall a couple of times.
- If you've got an exercise bike at home, pedal for five minutes while you're talking on the phone or waiting for the laundry to finish.

OFFICE WORKER
- Take the stairs — not the elevator.
- Walk during your lunch hour.
- Get up and go visit your co-workers instead of e-mailing them.
- Do stretching exercises at your desk.
- Have a walking meeting; meet with a co-worker to walk somewhere.
- Suggest an interoffice softball (or bowling or running) league.

WEEKEND WARRIOR
- Mow the grass with a push mower.
- Manually wash your car.
- Walk the dog daily.
- Be opportunistic. If you're watching your child's soccer game, walk around the field.
- Walk the golf course instead of using a cart.
- Schedule regular walks around your neighborhood with your kids, or hike the trails outside your town.

COUCH POTATO
- Stretch while you watch TV. Better yet, buy an exercise bike and pedal during TV shows.
- Ditch the remote and get up from the sofa to change the channel.
- Find a partner. Exercise can be more interesting if you chat away the time with a friend.
- Schedule dinner 30 minutes earlier and go for a walk afterward.
- Instead of heading for a snack during commercials, walk around the outside of your house five times.

TRAVELER
- Take a walk around the terminal while you're waiting for your flight.
- Do sit-ups, push-ups and stretching exercises in your hotel room.
- Book a room in a hotel with an exercise facility.
- Get up early and walk the neighborhood around your hotel.
- Schedule a business meeting at the local gym.

from osteoporosis to coronary artery disease.

If you have the following conditions, you might want to make allowances when devising your fitness routine:

Coronary artery disease
Regular exercise can help your heart pump blood more efficiently, improve your cholesterol levels and lower your blood pressure slightly. So why wouldn't you want to do it?

If you're worried about having a heart attack during exercise, remember that most heart attacks occur during rest, not activity. Of those who have heart attacks while exercising, most were sedentary or infrequent exercisers who started a program that was too vigorous for them. You will reduce your risk of a heart attack during rest by exercising.

You can minimize your risk and maximize the benefits of

Aches and pains
If you've been sedentary for a long time, you're bound to feel at least mild discomfort after starting any exercise routine. Rest assured, you probably haven't injured yourself. It's just your body going through a new challenge. Here's how to handle the pain:

- Get up and get going. Your muscles need gentle activity to enhance blood flow and promote healing within the muscle. Take a leisurely stroll, for example, or ride an exercise bike with no resistance.
- Choose acetaminophen, such as Tylenol or Panado, or take a nonsteroidal anti-inflammatory, such as aspirin or ibuprofen, with food to minimize stomach upset.
- Stretch your muscles after your initial workouts. Gentle stretching will reduce muscle soreness when you first start exercising.
- If you don't feel better within a few days, see your doctor, especially if the pain is beyond normal achiness, if a specific joint, such as your knee or ankle, is swelling, or if you must change what you normally do to compensate for the pain.

exercise by following the recommendations of your physician. Your doctor can give you a prescription for exercise, outlining how vigorous and how long. Start slowly. Then exercise regularly. Avoid intense competition and listen to your body. If you experience heart palpitations, lightheadedness or pain in your chest, jaw or arm, stop exercising immediately and call your doctor.

Diabetes

Exercise can lower your blood sugar and helps insulin work better. Plan your activity to fit around mealtimes and your medication dosage.

Try eating a small snack before you exercise, especially if it has been more than an hour since you last ate. Eat a small carbohydrate snack either before or during any mild to moderate exercise. Once you establish a regular exercise program, your doctor may need to lower the amount of insulin or oral medication you take.

Osteoporosis

Regular exercise is one of the best things you can do for osteoporosis because it builds muscle and helps maintain bone density. In fact, weight-bearing exercise may even increase bone density, which means your bones will grow stronger. In addition, by strengthening your muscles and bones, you can improve your balance and reduce the risk of falls and fractures.

Weight-bearing exercise is exercise that supports your body weight. Swimming, for example, is not a weight-bearing exercise.

Brisk walking can be an ideal exercise for osteoporosis because it's a weight-bearing exercise that you can do anywhere, with minimal risk of injury. If walking is painful, try riding a bike. The important thing is to exercise by putting weight on your bones and muscles while avoiding jarring maneuvers or activities that may contribute to a fall. You may even want to consider a low- to moderate-intensity weight-lifting program.

Arthritis

Although arthritis pain and stiffness may make you want to curl up under the electric blanket, using your joints during regular, appropriate exercise can help maintain good range of motion in your joints and may reduce pain. The best types of activity for arthritis seem to be walking, cycling, and swimming or water aerobics.

Start each session by warming up. Add time and intensity gradually. Don't overdo it. If you have severe pain, stop that particular exercise. Identify the time of day when joint pain is at its lowest and do your exercises then. Avoid high-impact exercise, and take a pain reliever if you need it.

Extreme obesity

In general, the greatest restrictions that extreme obesity imposes on activity come from other problems associated with excess weight. Although obesity makes it more difficult to move, which creates breathlessness and stress on underused muscles, excess weight can aggravate degenerative arthritis, make it harder to recover from surgery and increase susceptibility to infection.

Check with your doctor before starting an exercise program. Get a complete physical and explore activities that would provide the healthiest way for you to add appropriate and healthful movement to your life. Remember to start slowly and add repeated small amounts of activity. Find activities you can do, such as pedaling a stationary bike or a recumbent exercise bike, walking in water, or using an arm-exercise machine.

Start slowly, pick activities you enjoy and gradually build them into your life. You'll have a greater chance of sticking with it if you make physical activity a part of your lifestyle.

The family way

If you're adding physical activity to your life, congratulations. The health benefits will serve you well. But there's one way to extend those benefits even further, and that's by making sure your children understand the value of a fitness-oriented life.

Children are about six times more likely to be active when both parents exercise. That means if you exercise, your kids probably will, too. Developing a good physical fitness routine with your children helps them establish a pattern they will benefit from throughout their life — and pass along to their own children — and it gives you a way to add enjoyment to your own life at the same time.

It's only temporary

Everyone's been there. You're besieged with work, vacation or illness, and all those good exercise intentions fly right out the window. You're not alone. More than half the people who enroll in supervised exercise programs drop out within the first six months. How can you keep those little breaks in your physical routine from becoming permanent? Try these tips:

- Don't be too critical. Look upon every lapse as a learning experience. Remind yourself it's a temporary setback and not a catastrophe. It's just a momentary suspension of your program.
- Be realistic. Do you think you can exercise 2 hours a day 365 days a year? If this is your goal, you may be setting yourself up to fail. Instead, start with 30 minutes of activity 3 days a week and build on that.
- Continually plan. Think of ways to incorporate short periods of physical activity in your day even if you have a trip coming up or your workload increases. Planning may prevent relapse.
- Make it a priority. Exercise is just as important as anything else you do during the day.
- Get going. Do some kind, any kind, of physical activity today.

It's not difficult to instill an exercise mentality at home. Start by finding activities that everyone can do together. If you have infants or toddlers, invest in a stroller designed for jogging. If your children are preschoolers or school-aged children, plan regular walks to a nearby park or playground, enter an all-ages 5K fun walk for charity or explore the local hiking trails with a picnic lunch. For more structured fitness programs, check out your local

YMCA or other community organization. Many offer parent-child exercise classes and youth fitness programs in addition to those for adults.

Try some family brainstorming. What activities would appeal to both kids and adults? How will you make the time for family outings? Can you agree to spending more time outside for starters? Consider these other family activity tips:

- As a family, plan an activity at least three times a week for 20 to 30 minutes. This could be a session of basketball in the driveway, a backyard game of tag or a bike ride. If you can't block out 20 to 30 minutes at one time, break the time into 10-minute segments. But make sure it's fun.
- Set limits on the amount of time the kids can spend in front of the TV or computer — such as 1 hour a day or 10 programs a week.
- Incorporate more activity into everyday life. Walk to the store or park instead of driving. Walk up and down the sidelines at the soccer game instead of sitting in the stands.
- Make exercise enjoyable and varied. Remember that a lot of kids' games are exercise, so try to join in on some of their fun.
- Plan vacations and outings that involve physical activity: hiking, swimming, skiing or canoeing, for starters.
- Take it slowly if your family has been inactive.
- Talk to your children about the importance of fitness.

Taking the next step

You've decided to move beyond subtle increases in your daily activities. You want to devise the perfect workout. Where can you obtain the advice you need?

Health clubs deserve consideration. By shopping around, you can probably locate one near you where trainers will assess your physical fitness and recommend exercises most suitable to your lifestyle and interests. Joining a health club may also motivate you, since you've probably paid a hefty fee.

Here's what you can expect from a health club:

- Fitness on your level. If you're just starting a program, look for a fitness center where programs are geared for beginners. More advanced classes and experienced members, though, can also be an incentive as you learn.
- Certified staff members. Health and wellness instructors should be certified by the American College of Sports Medicine or the National Strength and Conditioning Association.
- Friendly employees. Do staffers smile and greet you? Do they get to know you — your likes, dislikes and habits? Do they offer regular tips and encouragement? You should expect interest and commitment from fitness center staffers.
- A clean, safe environment. Are the equipment and floors clean? Are staff members certified to give first aid and CPR? Are they continually tidying up and providing a safe exercise environment?
- The right atmosphere. Not all health clubs are filled with hard bodies. Take a look around the center. Will you want to visit this center regularly? Most reputable clubs will allow you to work out a time or two free before you join. Take advantage of trial opportunities.

Home alone

Health clubs are just one option. Working out at home has advantages, too. You won't have to wait in line to use exercise machines. You alone set the time for your workout. You choose your workout partners. But if you exercise at home, you may have to be more highly motivated to ignore distractions that will come your way, such as ringing phones, housework and drop-by visitors. The good news is that people who exercise at home are often more committed; they stick with their program and lose weight.

Before buying home fitness equipment, make sure you've carefully considered your own personality. If you've made exercise a habit and appreciate its benefits, then you're already ahead of the game. But if your well-meaning intentions of getting to the gym often fizzle, chances are good that you won't work out at home, either — and before long, you'll be selling that expensive stationary bike in your next garage sale.

Finding the ideal home equipment means determining what you most like to do. Next to lack of motivation, boredom probably kills more exercise programs than anything else. Ease into your home workout, try a number of different activities. If you've narrowed your preference to an activity such as walking, a treadmill may be a good investment.

Should you see your doctor?

Check with your doctor before starting any strenuous exercise program, especially if you've been inactive for a while. If you have additional health problems or are at risk of cardiovascular disease, take extra precautions before you begin. It's especially important to see your doctor if:

- You're a man age 40 or over, or a woman 50 or older, and you haven't had a recent physical examination
- You have diabetes, heart, lung or kidney disease
- Your blood pressure is 160/100 mm Hg or higher
- You have a family history of heart-related problems before age 55
- You're unsure of your health status
- You've previously experienced chest discomfort, shortness of breath or dizziness during exercise or strenuous activity

---

Crafting a plan

There are 3 main types of physical activity: aerobic, strength training and flexibility. These are explained in the sections that follow. You should include all 3 types in your program.

When planning your exercise program, consider that a typical session might include a 5-minute warm-up, 30 minutes of aerobic activity, and 5 to 10 minutes to cool down and stretch. Also consider 10 to 20 minutes of strength and balance exercises several times weekly.

At first, this may seem quite time-consuming, but look at it this way: It is one of the most important things you can do in your day.

You don't have to start out doing it all at once. Instead, figure the 1-hour workout is something to shoot for within perhaps 6 months of gradually increasing your exertions.

Aerobic exercise

Aerobic means "with oxygen," as opposed to anaerobic, "without oxygen." Aerobic workouts, such as walking and swimming, increase your breathing and heart rates. Anaerobic exercises, such as weight-lifting, work muscle groups.

While working out aerobically, you should be able to carry on a brief conversation without extra huffing and puffing. If you're out of breath, your body isn't getting the oxygen it needs to burn fat, but is relying instead on burning sugars. Exert yourself enough to know you're working, but you should also feel you could keep it up for quite a while.

In addition, aerobic activity doesn't have to be long, expensive or inconvenient. Short doses of exercise add up — and some people find that varying their activities makes it easier to stay interested in moving about.

Remember: Start slowly. Don't go for bursts of activity. Instead, build up gradually by adding several minutes a week to your aerobic activity. But keep at it! Consistency over time is vastly more important than a lot of temporary surges.

Exercises for aerobic fitness

How much and how often? It's best to exercise 30 minutes daily at a "moderate" to "somewhat strong" intensity (3 to 4 on the Perceived Exertion Scale — see page 118). Do a variety of lower- and upper-body exercises, such as walking, swimming or jumping rope. Extend the time you spend on aerobic exercise by 1- to 5-minute increments over a period of weeks or months. Increasing the time gradually minimizes your risk of injury.

Walking. The best way to start exercising is simply to walk. You don't need equipment; you don't have to learn techniques. In addition to the weight-loss benefits you'll gain from this aerobic activity, walking is good for your heart, lungs and bones.

Walking isn't just a way to break into exercising; it's also a means to stay fit and healthy for the long haul. If you're just starting out, begin by walking 10 minutes a day. Each week, increase the length of time you walk by 2 to 5 minutes, and keep adding increments until you can walk 45 minutes to an hour at a time.

How many calories?

How much energy will you burn? The figures below show the approximate calories expended hourly by 150- , 200-, and 250-pound persons:

Activity	150 lb.	200 lb.	250 lb.
Bicycling, 6 mph	240	312	384
Bicycling, 12 mph	410	534	660
Bowling	240	300	360
Calisthenics	300	360	420
Dancing	420	600	780
Jogging, 7 mph	920	1,230	1540
Jumping rope	750	1,000	1250
Running in place	660	962	1264
Running, 10 mph	1,280	1,664	2044
Swimming, 25 yds/min	275	358	441
Swimming, 50 yds/min	500	650	800
Tennis, singles	400	535	670
Walking, 2 mph	240	312	380
Walking, 3 mph	320	416	600
Walking, 4.5 mph	440	572	700

Eventually, you'll be able to walk at a brisk pace. If you're an experienced exerciser, you may want to swing your arms more as you go, to provide some upper-body movement and to increase the aerobic intensity.

Jogging. If you jog at about 8 miles an hour, you'll burn twice as many calories as you do when you walk. This means you can be more efficient with your exercise time. But there's a catch. Despite its aerobic benefits, jogging can be hard on your joints. The impact that comes from repetitious pounding can lead to injuries to your feet, ankles, knees and hips.

If this sounds like your kind of exercise, start slowly. Especially if you've been inactive for a while, try walking first. Once you can walk 2 miles in about 30 minutes, then you're ready to alternate jogging and walking, by jogging for 1 minute, then walking for another minute, and so forth.

Using the Perceived Exertion Scale

The Perceived Exertion Scale refers to the total amount of physical effort you experience during a physical activity, taking into account all sensations of exertion, physical stress and fatigue. When using the rating scale, don't become preoccupied with any one factor, such as leg discomfort or labored breathing, but try to concentrate on your total inner feeling of exertion.

For the activity to produce health benefits, you need to exert a "moderate" to "somewhat strong" effort. That means you'll need a 3 or 4 on the Perceived Exertion Scale. A "0" rating indicates a minimal level of exertion, such as sitting comfortably in a chair, while a "10" corresponds to a maximal effort, like jogging up a steep hill.

Remember that when you first start small amounts of activity, you will feel "moderate" to "somewhat strong." That's OK. The longer you keep at it, the more you'll be able to do.

0 Nothing at all

1 Very weak

2 Weak

3 Moderate

4 Somewhat strong

5 Strong

6 Stronger

7 Very strong

8 More difficult

9 Very difficult

10 Extremely difficult

To minimize potential muscle and joint discomfort, limit your sessions to three to four a week on alternate days. Jog at a comfortable pace and walk briskly, keeping within the guidelines of your perceived exertion and target heart rate range (see page 122).

Buy a good pair of running shoes. Also consider an elliptical running machine, which can provide a movement similar to jogging without the stress to your joints. Alternate jogging with gentler forms of exercise.

Bicycling. Bicycling is a great way to get aerobic exercise. And you don't have to ride outside all year. Consider a stationary upright or recumbent bicycle indoors for all-weather conditioning. When the weather's nice, consider making a bicycle ride a part of your weekend activities. Choose different trails in your area, or find off-the-beaten paths that will provide some scenery with your exercise.

Swimming. Exercising in the water is as close as you can get to a no-impact aerobic workout. Water provides 12 times the resistance of air, so you can get a good workout without risking joint damage. If you want to make this individual activity a group event, enroll in a water aerobics class.

Aerobic dance. Some people shy away from this activity because it's often done in group settings. But many health centers offer classes for the sweatshirt set. These programs are for people who need to start moving at a more basic level. If you're motivated by others — and by the energy of a class — this could be a great way to get your aerobic workout. You can also rent or buy aerobic exercise videos.

Ski machine. This gives an excellent overall workout, but it can be a difficult machine to start on. Your arms and legs move in rhythmic opposition, like walking. At first you may feel off-balance. You'll need to practice to achieve the smooth skiing motion that's required.

Elliptical cross-trainer. Providing a total upper and lower body workout, this aerobic machine offers the combined benefits of running, stair climbing, cycling and cross-country skiing in a single device. Like the ski machine, it encourages your arms and legs to move in an elliptical motion, and it's easy on your joints. The exercise is as natural as walking.

Strength and balance

Each year, between the ages of 30 and 70, you'll lose about 1 percent of your muscle strength, primarily through inactivity. That means you could be 40 percent weaker at 70 than you were at 30. Weight-lifting, also called strength or resistance training, can slow this process. Adding strength training to your activity mix will help you continue doing all the things you enjoy.

Working out with either free weights or on exercise machines is an excellent way to build lean-muscle mass because it simulates motions you make in day-to-day life, such as carrying boxes or lifting sacks of groceries — and makes these activities easier. When your muscles work against gravity, they grow stronger. Your bones become sturdier and more dense. Strength training, therefore, strengthens both your skeleton and the muscles that support it, which combats aging-related weaknesses and contributes to good balance.

Again, begin slowly. One set of 12 repetitions can be just as effective as doing three sets of four "reps." Consider finding a

Options, options

Wondering how to get your exercise? Whether you want to work on your upper or lower body, you have many indoor and out-door activity choices:

Upper-body workout activities
- Indoor: Push-ups, table tennis, kneading bread, vacuuming
- Outdoor: Archery, horseshoes, kayaking, fly fishing, canoeing

Lower-body workout activities
- Indoor: Basketball, hockey, ice skating, stair climbing, tread-mill, elliptical cross trainer
- Outdoor: Running, walking, bicycling, hiking, soccer, inline skating, downhill skiing, snowshoeing

Combination workout activities
- Indoor: Jumping jacks, jumping rope, volleyball, strength training or weight-lifting, rowing, tai chi, yoga, aerobic dance
- Outdoor: Badminton, cross-country skiing, football, tug of war, swimming, climbing, tennis, softball, soccer, gardening.

certified professional to teach you the right form, since improper technique is one of the leading causes of injury.

In sickness and in health
We've all heard the benefits of the buddy system. But one study found that people who exercise with a spouse are two to three times more likely to adhere to their workout program.

Work all the major muscle groups: abdominals, legs, chest, back, shoulders and arms. Make sure your workout is balanced, which means you should strengthen muscles on both sides of a joint equally. For example, work your triceps as well as your biceps, hamstrings (back of thigh) as well as quadriceps (front of thigh), and your back (latissimus dorsi) muscles as well as those of your chest (pectorals).

Not all strengthening exercises have to be done with weights. Exercises that use your body's own resistance to objects around you include push-ups against a wall, chair dips and standing squats.

Flexibility and stretching

Everyone has a different genetic set point for flexibility. No matter what your level, however, you can improve and become more flexible.

Although it's good to stretch before and after exercise, you might not have time to do both. Instead, start your exercise with a leisurely version of your preferred activity that day. If you are walking, for example, warm up with 5 minutes at a slower pace, then gradually build up speed. Stretch after you finish your walk. It's especially important to stretch when your muscles are warmed up, or after you've exercised.

When stretching, hold your stretches for 10 to 30 seconds. Don't bounce. Focus on the muscles you use most. If you play golf or racquet sports, for instance, concentrate on your shoulder muscles. If you walk or run, stretch your calf muscles, hamstrings and quadriceps. No matter what you do, keep your torso flexible by

Stop immediately

No matter what your workout routine, be sure to heed any warning signs that tell you to stop. If you feel tightness in your chest or are severely short of breath, for example, stop exercising and seek care immediately. Other sensations to watch for include chest pains; pain in your arms or jaw, especially on the left side; palpitations; or dizziness, faintness or feeling sick to your stomach.

stretching your back and chest muscles. A healthy spine is crucial to every activity, and you must keep it limber and strong.

At the end of every workout, be sure to take time to cool down for 5 to 10 minutes. To cool down, you can do more stretching exercises or, if you're walking, for example, simply slow your pace to a stroll.

Recording your progress

Consider keeping a record of your progress, because one of the best ways to change a habit is to keep track of it. The American Heart Association and other nonprofit groups offer their own versions of exercise diaries, but you can make your own. An exercise log will let you see what you've accomplished and help set your goals for the future.

After each exercise session, you might record:
• The date
• The activity (jogging, swimming, bicycling, etc.) and whether it's aerobic, strength training or flexibility.
• Your exercise heart rate. Immediately after you stop exercising, take your pulse for 10 seconds and multiply it by 6 to get your heart rate per minute. Your maximum heart rate is approximately 220 minus your age. Your "target heart rate" (the rate you should try for during your exercise regimen) is 50 percent to 70 percent of your maximum heart rate.
• The duration or extent of your activity. Simply record laps,

Lifestyle changes

I was a couch potato with an international reputation. Friends from coast to coast — and in Europe and Asia, too — knew that I would go to great lengths to avoid exercise, and that I was even proud of my slothful status.

Shortly after my 40th birthday, however, I realized my clothes seemed to have become tighter. When I caught a glimpse of myself in a full-length mirror shortly after a shower, I knew I had a problem.

My desk job required that I take decisive action. I wasn't going to lose 20 pounds with my daily activities, of which there were pitifully few. So, with my husband's encouragement, we joined a university recreation center less than a mile from our home.

We started getting up at 5:30 a.m. I would immediately dress in my workout togs, even though we would spend the next hour reading the newspaper and drinking coffee. That way, I had no excuses when the appointed time came to head to the gym.

My routine was simple. I walked around an indoor track every day, Monday through Friday, for 1 hour. At first, my pace was on the slow side, but as I saw other walkers speeding by, I learned to pick up my pace. I read a few books on walking and discovered that I'd do best if I could walk at least a 15-minute mile. It was hard, but I managed it within a month.

By the time I lost the 20 pounds, six months later, I knew I would be walking for the rest of my life. I realized that losing the weight was nice, but the overall health benefits were even better. I had more energy and more stamina than ever before, and my hips had slimmed down enough that I could wear the same size top and bottom — for the first time in my life.

As I've learned more about physical activity, I've added 15 minutes of weight lifting twice a week. When the weather gets nice, from March through October, I walk outside, sightseeing through the neighborhoods in our vicinity.

It's been nearly six years since I launched my fitness program, and it's one of the best decisions I ever made. I believe it has added years of health and enjoyment to my life.

Linda
Kansas City, Missouri

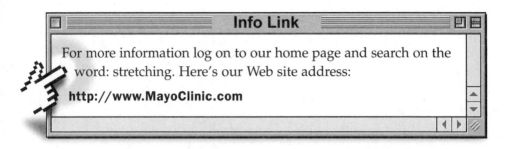

For more information log on to our home page and search on the word: stretching. Here's our Web site address:

http://www.MayoClinic.com

miles, kilometers, minutes, hours or any other meaningful measurement.

• Your mood. How did you feel before and after your workout? Was it your first workout in a week? How did you feel that day?

Recording your progress also makes exercise seem a more conscientious and committed part of your life. With a daily written chronicle of your improvement, you will be more motivated to continue. And that's the whole idea.

A new attitude

No matter what exercise you undertake, the important thing is just to get moving, then make it a regular habit. If you want to launch an hour-long structured exercise program that sends you out the door at 6:30 every morning, that's great. If you'd rather break up your activity into bite-sized pieces that you can nibble on throughout the day, that's fine, too.

Strive for an attitude that acknowledges physical activity as a building block of every weight-loss program and as a foundation for living a healthy life. As a well-known athletic shoe manufacturer has told us, "just do it." Nothing could be more apt when it comes to your ideal approach to physical activity.

Chapter 9

Changing attitudes and actions

- Changing your behavior requires a firm commitment.
- Short-term deprivation doesn't work.
- Long-term lifestyle changes do.
- Keep a food journal.
- Identify "triggers" that encourage you to eat.
- Plan carefully.
- Get the support you need.

Why do you eat the way you do? Why do you eat more than you need? Do you find yourself putting food into your mouth when you're not hungry? Well, you learned that behavior. The good news is, you can unlearn it.

The only proven formula for achieving and maintaining a healthy weight — eat less and move more — sounds easy. But anyone who's overweight and who has tried to follow the formula knows it's more challenging than it sounds. What gets in the way?

Many things, among them habits, emotions, needs, conditioned thinking and lack of awareness. It's those you need to target, not just what and how you eat, if you want to make lasting changes. Your eating behavior and your weight aren't isolated from the rest of your life. They're part of who you are. So you have to address all aspects of your lifestyle to make permanent changes.

Changing your lifestyle is more than choosing different foods and putting more activity into your day. It also involves changing your approach to eating and activity, which means changing how you think, feel and act. Sound tough? It is. It takes concentration, focus and effort. It requires a firm commitment. That's why achieving and maintaining a healthy weight are so challenging. But have faith. Research has demonstrated that a number of tools are effective in helping you change, and we're going to show you what those tools are and how to use them.

First, think this through

Here's a typical scenario: You get on the scale one morning and you're dismayed by the number, or you put on a pair of pants you haven't worn for a while, and they don't zip. Your first reaction is panic. "Oh my gosh," you think, "I've gained more weight." The panic is frequently accompanied by negative self-assessments: "I'm a blimp." "I have no willpower." "I'll never lose weight."

The panic and negative thoughts are then followed by one of two reactions. One is hopelessness. You go to the kitchen and, oversized serving spoon in hand, wrap yourself around a quart of Ben & Jerry's. "What's the use?" you ask yourself. "I'm destined to be fat."

The other reaction is fierce determination. You tell yourself you've had it. You're going to live on water and carrot sticks and walk 10 miles a day until you weigh what you weighed in college, by George.

Unfortunately, both reactions are equally self-defeating. Neither will result in any useful changes that lead to a healthy weight you can maintain. Both will leave you cranky. So what do you do?

If you're serious about reaching a healthy weight, then you can't just drastically cut your food intake, up your exercise and hope for the best. You need to approach losing weight as you would any significant, long-term achievement. You need to look at the obstacles you face and find ways around them. You have to set goals and figure out ways to meet them. You have to determine what help you need and from whom and figure out ways to get it. In other words, you need a plan.

When people start a weight-loss program, they frequently don't think through the long-term work and lifestyle changes that are involved. This lack of planning leads to dropout.

Unfortunately, dropout leads to more self-defeating attitudes and negative self-talk, which strengthens your belief that you just can't lose weight. And that reaction often sends you to — you guessed it — the refrigerator or pantry for comfort. Of course, you realize as soon as you've polished off a big snack, that's the worst thing you could do to yourself.

Before you jump headfirst into the deep end of the diet pool, ask yourself these questions: What's my motivation? How's my stress level? How's my life going in general? Let's look at each question more closely.

Motivation

Why do you want to lose weight? Try this: Make a list of all the benefits of weight loss, such as having more energy, improving your health, wearing clothes that fit better, feeling better about yourself. Write down everything you can think of.

Now write down all the obstacles, such as having to keep track of what you eat, having to find time to exercise, hating the feeling of being hungry or whatever you've experienced during weight-loss attempts in the past. Consider everything. For example, does being overweight make you feel safe in some way? Does it provide you with excuses not to do things you're afraid to do, such as getting a better job or pursuing a dream? Write down everything that comes to mind, no matter how trivial, far-fetched or silly it may seem.

Now look at which list is longer. You can increase your motivation for weight loss by making sure the positives outweigh the negatives. Designed for quitting smoking or problem drinking, this process calls for focusing on the benefits and finding solutions to the obstacles. It also works with weight loss.

For example: No time to exercise? Brainstorm some solutions. Perhaps you can get up 20 minutes earlier to take a 15-minute walk before breakfast. Take another before dinner, and you've worked 30 minutes of activity into your day. Or maybe you can use your lunch hour to get in some physical activity. (Don't groan at the thought of adding one more thing to your overloaded day. Think of how much better you'll feel. If your day is overflowing, then look for what you can cut out to make room for exercise.)

Perhaps an obstacle for you is that you buy sweets for your kids, and then you end up eating them yourself. (Be sure you're being honest with yourself. Whom are you really buying sweets for?) Perhaps you could convince your kids to eat healthier along with you so that you can replace their sweet snacks with fruit and other healthy choices. Or you could buy sweets you don't like. Or have someone in the family store them out of your sight. Whatever you do, keep reminding yourself that for every problem, there's a solution.

Another way to increase your motivation is to build your self-confidence. If you've failed to achieve your goals during previous weight-loss attempts, chances are you're asking yourself why it would be different this time. Focus on what did work in the past. Say you lost 10 pounds. What helped you do that? Did you follow a particular program? Cut down on your fat intake? Walk regularly with a friend?

Incorporate those proven elements into this attempt. It's important to look at your previous successes and build on them. After all, even if you gained the weight back, you still succeeded in losing it in the first place. Give yourself some credit, and go from there.

Stress level

If you just lost your job, are in the midst of a divorce or are caring for a sick parent, then this may not be the best time to try to make big changes. Everyone's life is stressful, but we all know that stress ebbs and flows. Some times are tougher than others. If you're coping with some of life's biggest challenges, you might be wise to postpone (notice we said postpone, not cancel) tackling weight loss until things ease up a bit. Achieving healthy weight takes concentration and energy. You may not have it to give just now, and that's OK.

Life in general

Again, if your life feels out of whack, then this may not be the time to try to lose weight. Don't try to trick yourself into thinking you can wait until everything's calm, because life is never calm, but do wait until things are ticking along pretty normally for you. You could use this time, however, to plan your weight-loss approach.

Another caveat: Once you've embarked on your healthy weight effort, don't use life's ups and downs as an excuse to quit. If you get hit with the unexpected at work or at home (and you can count on it), then cut yourself some slack if you need to, but stay with your program. For instance, you could determine to maintain your current weight loss but not work at losing any more until the crisis passes. Whatever you do, sustain your motivation and keep sight of what's working for you.

Know thyself

For your plan to work, you need to understand what makes you tick, particularly in regard to your eating habits. One of the best ways to do that is to keep a journal. Unlike the food record described in Chapter 7 (see page 90), the purpose of this journal is to show you not just what you eat, but when and why.

Yes, keeping a journal takes some effort. But studies show that it's one of the success tools used by people who achieve and maintain a healthy weight. It's so effective, in fact, that several studies have shown that simply keeping a journal causes some people to reduce their food intake, probably by increasing their awareness of their eating behavior.

Perhaps more important, however, is that keeping a journal can show you what triggers your eating and why you eat when you're not hungry.

Keep a journal
Here's how it works. Carry a small notebook with you. Every time you put something in your mouth, write down what you ate. If you want to combine your journal with your food record, record portion sizes in ounces, cups, teaspoons, and so on. You don't have to weigh and measure everything you eat and drink. Just pay

attention and estimate serving sizes (see page C5).

That's not all. Write down the date (day and month), the time, where you ate (in your car, at your desk), how you felt (bored, anxious, guilty, rushed), whom you were with and how fast you ate (slow, moderate or fast). Also write down — and this is very important — what triggered your eating. Did someone offer you something? Were you hungry? Were you angry? Did you pass a bakery? Then assess how hungry you were. Be honest. That doughnut might have tasted fabulous, but did your stomach call for it (true hunger) or just your mouth (mouth hunger or craving)?

Leave room for all nine categories in your journal:
• Date
• Time
• Place
• Feelings
• Triggers
• With whom
• What you ate (including portion size and number of servings)
• Hunger
• Rate of eating

For a few days at least, try not to let your recording what you consume alter your eating patterns. After a few days, you should be able to see those patterns. Maybe every time you get angry or upset you find yourself reaching for cookies. Perhaps you can't resist the sight or smell of tempting food, no matter how recently you've eaten. Or perhaps you're afraid to hurt people's feelings, so whenever someone offers you food, you take it even if you don't want it. Whatever your patterns, once you become aware of them, you can work on changing them.

How to change

We tend to be comfortable with our habits and patterns of behavior. That means everybody resists change.

Think about how people reacted in your workplace or some organization to which you belong the last time someone tried to institute a change. Even if the change was ultimately for the better, people probably grumbled about it.

Some openly resisted, no doubt. Maybe a few quit, rather than making the necessary adjustments.

Change is hard, but not impossible. We all underestimate our ability to change. Take a small example: Many people have switched from drinking whole milk to skim. Maybe they tapered off gradually, from whole to 2 percent to 1 percent to skim. Or maybe they cut from whole to skim in one fell swoop. Either way, they made what they thought was an impossible change, and now that they're used to skim milk, whole milk tastes too thick and rich.

Now take a moment to think about some of the big changes you've faced in your life — getting married, moving, starting a new job, whatever — and how you adjusted. You got through it. Focus on the strengths you relied on then, because they're going to be helpful now.

Use your food journal to figure out what you need to change. Before we talk about specific change methods, take this to heart. Repeat it as a mantra or write it down and put it where you'll see it throughout the day: The first rule of change is to take it slowly. You're trying to develop a new lifestyle. It's not a race, and it can't happen overnight.

Don't use numbers on the scale as a measure of your success. You can't control the scale. You can, however, control what you eat and your activity level. So concentrate on those actions as your goal. Take one day at a time. Keep your motivation sharp and focus on feeling healthier and having more energy.

Another idea you need to imprint on your brain before you start: You will backslide. It's inevitable, and it's OK. There will be days when you eat more or move less than you intended. The important thing is not to use it as an excuse to give up. Have a plan for such occasions. You couldn't walk today because you ran out of time or the weather was bad? Don't beat yourself up. Add 5 minutes a day to your walks until you've made up the time.

You ate a slice of pizza you hadn't planned on? So what? Think about what triggered your unexpected eating and try to learn from it, then cut back a bit on your calories for a time to make up the difference. Let it even out over the week. Keep in mind that lean people don't eat the same amount of food every day. They maintain a balance over time.

Anticipate having a lapse. Plan for how you'll recover from an overeating episode. Know that you're not going to be perfect.

Trigger-happy

It's time to tackle those habits that need changing. Study your journal to see what trips you up. A good place to start is to look at your cues, or what triggers your eating (see page 41). If your diary shows that you eat mostly from hunger, then you've got a strength to build on. But if you see that you eat whenever you're happy, sad, frustrated or angry, whenever you pass a bakery or vending machine, or when anyone offers you food, then you need to work on stimulus control.

Certain situations or places may have become linked with eating in your mind, so when you're in those situations or places, you automatically eat. For instance, if you always find yourself munching a bag of potato chips when you watch the late news, then watching the news is linked with eating potato chips.

So what can you do about it? You have to break the link between whatever triggers your eating and your reaction to it. Depending on your triggers, you can accomplish stimulus control through a number of strategies.

The Zen of eating. Always eat mindfully. Pay attention to what you put in your mouth, and be aware of every bite. To accomplish mindful eating, you can't be doing anything else at the same time. Don't read. Don't watch TV. Just eat. Savor your food. Really taste it, smell it and feel its texture. Remember, eating is supposed to give you pleasure, not just fuel your body.

If you've ever consumed the better part of a quart of ice cream without even realizing you were eating, you know what it's like to eat without awareness. There's nothing pleasurable about it, and you feel sheepish (not to mention piggish) afterward. Eating with awareness will take some practice, but it's well worth the effort. Not only will you enjoy your food more, you'll be satisfied with less.

Time is of the essence. If your food diary shows that you eat many times during the day, having a schedule could give you a sense of control. It doesn't have to be the traditional three square meals. Create a schedule that's convenient for you, one that will enable you to eat when you're hungry. You can build some flexibility in by giving time frames, such as breakfast between 7 and 7:30 a.m., rather than static times.

You might find that eating three meals and two snacks works for you. Or perhaps six minimeals would suit your lifestyle better. The important thing is to set a schedule and stick with it. (But don't go more than 4 or 5 hours without eating or you could become ravenous.) If you find yourself craving something 20 minutes before your scheduled snack time, see whether you can wait it out. You might not even be hungry by the time the appointed hour rolls around. If you can't wait, at least have a healthful snack to start your meal.

Plan, plan, plan. At least a day in advance, plan what you'll eat the next day. What you eat will depend on how many calories you've decided you need to lose weight and the eating program you're following. But planning ahead and having the ingredients on hand will help keep you from grabbing a slice of leftover pizza when you arrive home hungry at dinnertime.

In the same vein, packing your lunch, snacks or even your breakfast to take to work will save you from relying on unhealthful vending machine or fast-food fare and from making impulsive food choices. It may sound time-consuming, but once you get in the habit of brown-bagging, you may even find it saves you time because you don't have to seek out food during the day.

Of course, the best plans can go astray. A good rule of preparedness is always to have something healthful to munch on, such as low-fat popcorn, cut-up veggies or fruit. That way, if an unexpected deadline keeps you working through your lunch hour, or you're on an airplane at dinnertime (forget the skimpy bag of peanuts), you'll always have something healthful to eat in an emergency.

Find your place. When you're eating at home, select one place for that activity, preferably at a dining table. Set the table, even if you're eating alone. Make it as pleasant as possible. And remember to pay attention to your food and not to do anything else while you eat. By eating in one place, you begin to associate that place and that place only with eating. If you never eat in the recliner while watching TV, then you're not as likely to get a sudden craving for cherry pie when you sit in the recliner or turn on the television. It's that simple. And that difficult. You have to break the ties that bind (and stuff) you.

Nix the junk. You might trick yourself into believing that bag of chocolate-covered peanuts you just tossed into your shopping cart is for the kids, but once it's in the house, can you resist? Do yourself and your kids a favor. Don't bring food into the house that doesn't contribute to everyone's health.

That doesn't mean you have to give up sweets. Plenty of foods that can satisfy a sweet tooth and provide needed nutrients. If you have time, look for recipes in cookbooks that emphasize low-fat and healthy. *The Mayo Clinic Williams-Sonoma Cookbook* is a good place to start, and your local bookstore has many others. Or shop in stores that offer nutritious alternatives to the standard high-fat, low-fiber, sugary concoctions that line the typical supermarket shelves. Beware, however, of low-fat baked goods and other low-fat products. They often have as many or more calories and more sugar than their higher-fat counterparts.

Keep in mind that as you practice your new eating habits, your tastes will change. You acquired your taste for prime rib, but believe it or not, you can unacquire it. Foods that once seemed dreamy eventually may taste too sweet or fatty. At the same time, you may discover that a parfait glass filled with peak-of-the-season berries topped with just a dollop of fat-free sour cream and a sprinkle of cinnamon sugar is your new idea of heaven on earth.

Shop from a list. This will keep you from impulsively or mindlessly slam-dunking that bag of potato chips into your cart. It also goes with planning ahead. Along those lines, don't shop when you're hungry, because you'll be tempted to grab anything that looks even vaguely appetizing. And while you're at it, read labels. Don't assume something's good for you because it's low fat. Check the sugar content, the calories and the sodium. If it has more chemicals than real food in it, do you really want it in your body?

Out of sight, out of mind. Store tempting food where you can't see it, especially if your diary reveals your eating is prompted by visual cues. Put it at the back of the cupboard or refrigerator, where it won't catch your eye every time you open the door.

Leave it, don't love it. Brace yourself for a shock: No matter what your parents told you when you were growing up, you don't have to finish the food on your plate. Even if you dished out what you consider to be a reasonable portion for yourself, how do you know before you start eating how much food you'll need to satisfy your hunger? And if someone dished it out for you, then how in the world would that person know how much food you need? Eat slowly, savor every bite, and stop when you're pleasantly full but not stuffed.

If you belong to the clean-plate club, start by leaving a dab of food at every meal just to signal your brain that it's OK. As you become more adept at identifying when you're hungry and when you're satisfied, it will become easier to take less food in the first place, and to leave food you don't want. Keep in mind that eating to the point of feeling stuffed is likely to trigger old feelings of guilt and negative self-thoughts about being out of control.

Strictly from hunger. Eating is comforting, so many people reach for food when they really want something else. Food can loom large when you're tired or thirsty, when you're lonely or sad, when you're angry or frustrated. Unfortunately, eating can't satisfactorily meet any need besides hunger. And eating for any other reason will almost certainly make you take in more calories than you need.

If you've been ignoring your hunger signals for a time and eating for other reasons, you may need to figure out what hunger feels like to you. Don't eat for a few hours and see how you feel. If what you're feeling isn't hunger, don't try to comfort yourself with food. If you're tired, then rest or meditate. If you're thirsty, drink a glass of water. If you're anxious, do some deep breathing, soak in a hot bath or take a walk. Stop making eating your all-purpose response. If you're not sure whether you're hungry, wait 15 to 30 minutes and see how you feel. Here's a clue: If you can't decide what you want to eat, chances are you're not hungry.

Gather the troops. One thing your food diary won't reveal is how helpful support can be as you go through the process of making the necessary changes to achieve your healthy weight. Be careful whom you enlist. We all have our own agendas, and they're not always conscious. So not everyone in your circle of friends and loved ones will be happy that you're losing weight. Pick a person or people you know want only the best for you and will encourage you.

The ideal support person might be a partner in your weight-loss effort, someone who also is trying to lose weight. Or it could be your spouse, co-worker or friend. Some people fare better with professional support, such as from a dietitian or personal trainer. Others like the group support they get from organizations such as Weight Watchers or Overeaters Anonymous.

Then there are people who like to work alone and don't want to ask for anyone's help. Do whatever works for you, but keep in mind that different approaches fit different needs.

Consider behavior modification. This involves examining the factors that lead to obesity (whether it's overeating or lack of physical activity), then alleviating or modifying these factors. The various treatment components of behavior modification programs include self-monitoring (recording your behaviors), stimulus control (restricting your external conditions), contingency management (rewarding appropriate behaviors), changing behavior directly (changing the way you act), and cognitive-behavior modification (changing the way you think).

How would this apply to you? One important key to self-monitoring, for example, is tracking everything you eat. People who keep dietary records are more successful at losing weight initially and maintaining it for the long term. A well-established behavior treatment program called LEARN — an acronym for lifestyle, exercise, attitudes, relationships and nutrition — may help you put this into practice. You can find out more about it on pages 138-139 and at www.learneducation.com.

Getting unstuck

If you're following the suggestions but still find yourself stuck in old patterns, you need to figure out what's keeping you immobile. We work to keep things the same. If you disturb the balance you created, such as by losing weight, then the balance will tend to right itself and return to business as usual. Which means you eventually regain the weight and return to the habits that caused you to be overweight in the first place. The trick is to disturb the balance in ways that create a new equilibrium when it rights itself.

The way to do that, according to a theory developed at Harvard University, is to challenge your big assumptions. Those are the things you think of as truth but are really just assumptions you make. Your perspective is not the truth. If you assume the world is flat, then you'll never venture far for fear of falling off.

Say, for instance, that you tell yourself you're destined to be overweight because you were born into an overweight family. Or that you've never been athletic, so you couldn't possibly sustain a workout program. Those are assumptions, not truths. You have to recognize your assumptions and examine them. Here's how:

- First, identify one of your big assumptions.
- Spend some time thinking about how your assumptions serve you. What does or doesn't happen when you accept your assumptions as gospel? What happens when you accept that they're merely assumptions?
- Be alert to anything that might disturb your big assumption. If you think you can't lose weight, then you lose 10 pounds, how does that affect your "truth"?
- Examine your assumption. How long has it been around? Where did it come from?
- Test the assumption in safe ways.

That means that you need to make changes slowly. Take small steps. Listen to yourself as you go. What are your thoughts and feelings as you discover that your assumption isn't truth? Are you relieved? Scared? Anxious? Don't ignore your feelings. Talk them over with a friend or counselor. Write about them in a journal. There are wonderful benefits to achieving and maintaining healthy weight. There are also potential drawbacks.

The drawbacks can be large or small. A large drawback could be that your extra weight makes you feel safe by protecting you from unwanted sexual attention. Or maybe you hide behind it for other reasons. If so, consider talking to a counselor who specializes in psychologic issues related to weight. Remember, every problem has a solution.

Deprivation is a no-no

In Chapter 6, you learned about healthy eating. Chapter 7 showed you how to develop a food plan and Chapter 8 told you how to incorporate activity into your daily life. By trying different things, you should be discovering new, healthy, pleasurable ways of eating and finding activities you enjoy.

Deriving pleasure from your new lifestyle is not just a pleasant bonus. It's vital to your success. If you're just gritting your teeth and tolerating the changes you've made, then chances are they won't last. If you think of yourself as being on a diet, then eventually you're likely to go off it and end up back where you started.

To reach your healthy weight and maintain it, you have to see the changes you're making as positive. A negative experience is something to get through as quickly as possible. Deprivation is no fun. That's why it's so important to take your needs into account and not try to follow an inflexible, one-size-fits-all plan.

Say you love hot fudge sundaes. Now that you're changing your eating habits, you tell yourself you can't have any. One day you get a craving for one. You dutifully munch on carrot sticks to squelch the craving, but they don't help. So then you start looking for other substitutes. You try fat-free yogurt, move on to low-fat ice cream with chocolate syrup and work your way up to a bag of chocolate chips. You've just engaged in a full-fledged binge. Chances are you're feeling stuffed and guilty and, worst of all, you still want a hot fudge sundae.

Or maybe for you deprivation doesn't lead to bingeing. Maybe it just leads to resentment. Eventually you'll find yourself living for the day when you can eat your favorite dessert again. When would that be? When you go off your diet, of course. Wrong script.

What would happen if, rather than making certain foods off-limits, you allow yourself to have them occasionally, accounting for them in your total intake? What if, on those occasions, you get the best hot fudge sundae you can lay your hands on, eat it as slowly and as mindfully as possible and stop when your craving is satisfied? You just might find that by savoring your favorite treat, paying attention to every spoonful, you only need a few bites.

Sound impossible? Try it. In *The LEARN Program for Weight Control*, a behavioral program for doctors to use with their patients who want to achieve healthy weight, authors Kelly Brownell, Ph.D., and Thomas Wadden, Ph.D., write about a woman named Ginny, who discovered she could have her ice cream and eat it too.

Ginny loved ice cream and ate a bowl every night. She was told to count her bites and note her pleasure in each. Ginny found that she averaged 16 bites. The first four were delicious, she paid little attention to the middle 10 and refocused her attention on the final few. Thanks to her new-found awareness, Ginny discovered she could cut out the middle ten bites. Remarkable. Simply by paying attention, she cut out more than half the fat and calories and heightened the pleasure.

Accentuate the positive

Rather than focusing on what you can't eat, focus on what you can. Look at what new tastes you can discover that will enhance your health. If, for example, you've never been much of a fruit eater, experiment with adding different fruits to your menus. Add blueberries to your cereal in the morning (try frozen or dried if fresh aren't available). How about some mango or peach slices on whole-wheat toast with peanut butter and honey? Toss some mandarin orange slices and raisins into a salad.

Flip through cookbooks and cooking magazines devoted to healthy cooking, such as *Vegetarian Times* and *Cooking Light*. No time to cook? That's no excuse. Today's recipes often are designed with quick and easy preparation in mind. Many cookbooks even note how much time the recipes require. By experimenting with new foods and new combinations, not only are you bound to find some tastes you love, thereby increasing your eating pleasure, but you'll also increase the variety of nutritious foods in your eating plan. And variety is very important in getting adequate nutrition and combating taste bud boredom.

Again, keep in mind that tastes are acquired. Eventually, your taste buds will adjust to your new style of eating. You'll like foods you never thought you would, and you may find some of your old favorites less appealing.

Pay attention, also, to how foods make you feel. Eating nutritious foods should give you more pep, not bog you down. If you eat a candy bar in midafternoon, then watch how your energy flags after a while. What happens after you eat some fruit and plain yogurt or cut-up veggies and salsa? Feel the difference? You might even get into the habit of asking yourself this: "Will what I'm about to put in my mouth contribute to my good health or simply add calories?" If it's just calories, then why eat it? Unless it's something you dearly love, skip it. If you dearly love it, then have just a bit. Your body will thank you.

Time is on your side

If you hop on the scale every morning and anxiously judge your success by how far it's moved, then you're setting yourself up for failure. First of all — and we can't emphasize this enough — change takes time. Second of all, if you're only focusing on pounds lost, then you're missing out on all the wonderful things your new lifestyle is doing for you, including the health benefits of your weight loss and increased activity, having more energy and feeling better about yourself.

Take your physical activity, for example. You get so much more out of being active than just burning calories. For one thing, once your body gets used to it, movement feels good. Your body was designed to move, not to sit all day. Being a couch potato drains you until you feel, well, half-baked.

Getting yourself to move also feels good because you know you're doing something positive and self-nurturing. Physical activity counteracts depression and relieves stress. It can help you sleep better. And studies show that most people who achieve and maintain healthy weight do it through a combination of changing their eating habits and adding activity to their day.

To get and keep yourself moving, you have to pick activities you enjoy. Walk, bike, swim, dance, hike in the woods. Hate exercise? Then create opportunities to engage in lifestyle activities, such as mowing the lawn, taking the stairs instead of the elevator, digging in the garden. The choices are endless. Find a partner. Listen to music. Do whatever moves you (pun intended).

If you've been sedentary, then set small achievable goals. Here are some ideas for keeping yourself motivated:

- Keep a log of your progress, recording either time spent or distance covered.
- Make a contract with yourself and put it in writing. Keep it where you can see it.
- Find a coach. If you can't afford a personal trainer, ask a friend to work out with you or to monitor your progress and encourage you.
- Reward yourself with something that matters to you every time you reach a goal.
- Set a regular time for your physical activity so that it becomes habit.
- Meditate while you move. You'll pack extra benefits into the same amount of time, practice your mindfulness and add a whole new dimension to your activity. There are a number of books on the subject, such as *The Spirited Walker: Fitness Walking for Clarity, Balance and Spiritual Connection,* by Masters champion fitness walker Carolyn Scott Kortge (HarperCollins, 1998).
- Develop positive self-statements or affirmations. Repeat them to yourself daily or type them and post them where you'll see them regularly. An example would be, "I'm getting stronger and better every day," or that old standby, "Every day in every way, I'm getting better and better." Create

affirmations that speak to you. Then repeat them until you mean them.

• Cut yourself some slack when necessary. Even champion athletes have days when working out seems like pure drudgery. Some days you're just plain tired. This isn't boot camp. As long as you know you're not using your tiredness as an excuse to quit, it's OK to take a day off now and then. Or you could try giving yourself 5 or 10 minutes to get into your regular workout. If, after the allotted time, you still feel awful, take the day off and try again tomorrow. The more you call the shots on your food and activity plan, the more you'll make it your choice and the less likely you are to rebel against it.

Put your whole self in

Remember the hokey pokey, the silly dance you did as a kid? You put different parts of yourself into the circle until, at the end, you put your whole self in. Putting your whole self in is what you have to do to achieve and maintain healthy weight. There will be days when you feel like pulling your whole self out. Know that from the start. On those days, be prepared to put yourself right back in again and shake it all about. Change is like that, especially the shaking up part. And like the hokey pokey, it can also be fun and rewarding.

If it helps, think of the changes you're making as a dance. You're learning new steps as you choreograph a new life for yourself, one that leads to better health and more self-confidence. One that leads to achieving your goals. Sometimes you'll trip over your own toes. Or you'll get so frustrated, you'll decide you're never going to get the hang of it. Then one day, you'll find yourself gliding along gracefully, and you'll realize it was worth all the time and effort. That doesn't mean you'll never trip again, but by then you'll know how to recover and move on.

Change is hard, but change is definitely possible. Just remember, put your whole self in. And when you start to feel a little too shaken all about, stop to analyze your feelings, talk to your support

No challenge too great

I have struggled with severe obesity for fifty years. I have tried just about everything. I've done Weight Watchers, Nutri-System, Overeaters Anonymous, TOPS. I've taken more kinds of diet drugs than I care to remember. I've been on the Atkins Diet, liquid diets, single-food diets. The only consistent thing was the results — dramatic initial weight loss followed by even more dramatic weight gain. I'd gain back all that I had lost and 5 to 20 pounds extra. I stayed around 300 pounds most of my adult life, ranging from 225 to around 400.

In 1997, physicians at the Mayo Clinic told me my life was now in danger from the severe obesity and I needed to make serious lifestyle changes. I told them I was 55 years old and couldn't imagine why I would have more success now than I ever had. I thought it was better that I just maintain at 330. But, the truth is, my body was breaking down. I had high blood pressure, elevated cholesterol and degenerative arthritis so severe I was a candidate for a knee replacement.

The doctors and registered dietitians at the Clinic worked with me to develop a low-fat, low-calorie diet tailored to my needs and tastes I could use as a guide for permanent change. They met with me regularly, offering support and guidance.

I significantly changed the way I prepare and eat food. I use fat-free dairy products. I spray my toast with butter-flavored Pam. I eat lots of fruits and vegetables and get my animal protein from seafood and bison, which is remarkably low in calories and fat. I keep a food record and turn it in to my dietitian for review. I don't eat at buffets. I do send extra food back to the kitchen so it's not there on my plate calling me.

In the first three months, I lost thirty-five pounds. At that point I added exercise to my regimen, just arthritis water classes at first. Gradually, I moved to land-based exercises including an elliptical trainer, recumbent bicycle and treadmill in addition to weights.

Gradually adjusting to a 1400-calorie diet, I lost 184 pounds in a two-year period and have been in maintenance for one and a half years. I weigh 150 pounds and love it. My BMI has gone from 58 to 25. My dress size has gone from a snug 32 to a comfortable 10.

Cynthia
Wichita, Kansas *Cynthia*

person, write in your journal — whatever helps you steady yourself and get back into the dance. Then take a deep breath, give yourself a well-deserved pat on the back and continue. You can do it.

Chapter 10

When the going gets tough

- **Expect a challenge.**
- **There's a solution to every problem.**
- **Get up after you fall.**
- **Never give up.**

Y ou've made the necessary lifestyle changes to reach a healthy weight. You're humming along on your new plan, feeling good about yourself, when BAM! something gets in your way. Maybe you've hit a plateau where for several weeks you see no results, or maybe some life crisis rears its ugly head and you revert to old behaviors. You find yourself scarfing unwanted potato chips from the bag, hating yourself and feeling powerless to stop. You panic, afraid that you'll undo all your good efforts and that your hard work will be for naught.

Calm down. Breathe. Use this as an opportunity to strengthen and reinforce your problem-solving skills and your resolve. Remember, we told you you'd have setbacks. They're normal and, more important, unavoidable. How you deal with them can make all the difference between success and failure. The crucial thing to remember is, you can deal with them.

Let's look at how.

Forming good habits

Habits are tenacious. You've worked hard for months to overcome the ones that contribute to your being overweight. You've kept a food journal, stopped eating mindlessly in front of the TV and established a routine of walking every evening. In other words, you've formed new good habits to replace the old bad ones. So one day, when you find yourself in your recliner during your walking time, watching a favorite TV program while devouring slices of deep-dish pizza with extra cheese, you have to ask yourself, "What happened?"

Merriam Webster's Collegiate Dictionary, Tenth Edition, defines habit in a number of ways, including "a behavior pattern acquired by frequent repetition or physiologic exposure that shows itself in regularity or increased facility of performance," "an acquired mode of behavior that has become nearly or completely involuntary" and "the prevailing disposition or character of a person's thoughts and feelings; mental makeup." In other words, your habits are a part of you, and you acquired them over a lifetime. They're automatic; most of the time, you perform habitual actions without thought. No wonder they're tenacious. What's a few months of new behavior compared to a lifetime of habit?

Don't despair. Habits are stubborn, not invincible. Think about a particular habit you want to change and try to remember how it started. For example, Janet (not her real name) used to come home from high school, grab a spoon, open the freezer, which was on the bottom of the refrigerator, plop down on the floor, pull the lid off the ice cream and eat herself into oblivion. It was a way of calming herself, of soothing the stress of a challenging day and making the transition from school to home. Is it any wonder that today, at age 50, when she feels stressed, she pulls out a spoon and a container of ice cream and digs in?

With her behavior, Janet developed a belief that she wasn't even aware of. She believed she needed the ice cream to be able to calm herself down enough to focus on her homework. For her, this belief was truth. Remember the big assumptions from Chapter 9? Those are the beliefs you hold that you think of as truth when they're really just your take on something. Chances are, if you examine your habits, you'll find a big assumption underlying each one.

When your beliefs and your habits support helpful, healthy behavior, they serve you well. But the ones that keep you stuck doing things that aren't good for you or that don't allow you to achieve your goals — well, it's time to give those the old heave-ho.

As you've experienced, knowing what you should do doesn't hold a lot of sway over habits. Habits are too tough for those puny, little "shoulds." For instance, we all know people, experts in their field, such as medical professionals, who smoke, who give advice but don't follow it themselves. If you know you should, say, move your body for 30 minutes a day, but you tell yourself you can't possibly spare that much time or you don't have that much energy or you can't imagine what difference it will make anyway, you've set up an internal conflict that will most likely keep you from being physically active, at least with any consistency. The beliefs underlying your habit of not moving are not at all puny. They're entrenched.

Even if you think the reason you can't get out to walk is physical (you're too tired) or social (your friend wants you to go shopping) or environmental (it's too cold outside), chances are it's the underlying belief that's causing you to respond to those behavioral triggers. So where should you look if you want to change your behavior? Examine your beliefs. We'll show you how.

Another thing you need to keep in mind when trying to change a habit is that it fulfills a need. For Janet, the ritual of eating ice cream after school soothed her after a stressful day. If you want to change the habit, you have to consider the need it addresses and find another way to meet it.

To change a habit, you can't just replace it with a new one. You have to change the belief that supports the habit, and you have to fill the need the habit meets. That's why, even though you've been practicing new habits for a time, you may revert to old ways when stressed or challenged. The old ways are automatic. They're learned behavior, and they're comfortable and comforting in some way.

The good news is they can be unlearned and replaced with new ways of behaving that also provide comfort.

Beliefs in action

Say you think you're destined to be fat. And you also believe that if you could only be thin, you'd be happy. Put those two beliefs together, and what have you got? The belief that you're destined to be unhappy.

Still, hope springs eternal, so you go on diet after diet. You lose weight, only to hit a plateau or a challenge that bounces you back to your old habits. You regain the weight, and, of course, you're miserable. Not only have you reinforced your belief that you're destined to be fat and unhappy, you've made failing at achieving and maintaining a healthy weight into a habit.

What would happen if you changed those underlying beliefs? True, it's easier said than done. But what would happen if you tried? Here's what you'd have to change:

- "I'm destined to be overweight" becomes "I can develop new eating and activity habits that will help me achieve and maintain a healthy weight."

- "If I were thin, I'd be happy" becomes "I need to look at what's making me unhappy now and make the changes necessary to gain satisfaction from my life. I need to learn to like and accept myself regardless of my weight, and find other ways to meet my needs than through food." To do all that, maybe you need professional help, such as therapy or a support group. Or perhaps you just need to keep a journal of your thoughts to become aware of the belief and stop it whenever it enters your head. Only you can judge.

As for the habit of going on and off diets, this entire book addresses how to replace that behavior with healthier approaches. But do be aware that it might have become a habit for you in and of itself. No matter how hard you try to make healthy lifestyle changes, if you have at the back of your mind that you'll fail because you always have, then root that nasty little saboteur out and bring it to the forefront. Keeping it in your awareness and telling yourself it isn't true anymore will help you get past it. This is a new day and a new you.

Remember Tinker Bell? She told Peter Pan that every time someone says he or she doesn't believe in fairies, another fairy dies.

Tinker Bell was saved from the brink of death by belief. True, it's just a fairy tale, but fairy tales represent universal truths. Belief is powerful. Examine your beliefs and change the ones that are keeping you stuck. Use affirmations, use self-talk, go into therapy, enlist the help of friends and family to get you back to life. You're worth it.

Most of all, believe in yourself.

Get real

Sometimes the tenacity of habits reflects a fundamental problem with what you're trying to achieve. Reconsider the goals you set for yourself going into this change process. Are you trying to achieve healthy weight for the right reasons? Are you doing it for yourself or because of some outside pressure?

Research suggests that you can change your behavior and make the changes stick if the change is autonomously motivated, meaning you're doing it for yourself. The theory proved true for 128 people on a very-low-calorie diet whom researchers followed throughout a 6-month weight-loss program and for nearly 2 years after. Those who scored high on a test of autonomous motivation were more likely to stay in the program, lose weight and maintain their weight loss than those who were doing it for someone or something else.

As important as having the right motivation is making a commitment to yourself. This is serious business. Say it out loud, tell loved ones, write it down. Do whatever makes it real for you. People who achieve healthy weight and maintain it make a commitment at the start.

After you make the commitment, ask yourself whether you've set a realistic weight-loss goal, and do you believe it's a good one? Maybe you told yourself you'd be happy to lose a half-pound a week, but you find that pace agonizingly slow. You want results, and you want them now. In that case, you can reassess your program, try to cut your food intake, and increase your activity level until you're losing 1 to 2 pounds a week, which is still an acceptable rate of loss. But first ask yourself whether eating less and moving more would increase your motivation or ultimately make your goals harder to achieve.

Remember, too, that even if you lose weight faster, you'll still encounter weeks of no weight loss and probably weeks when you gain a bit because of your body's natural fluctuations. So maybe you need to shift your focus.

Keep your eyes on the prize, and remind yourself that the changes you've made are for your lifetime. This isn't a diet you'll be going off when you achieve your goal. Yes, you can probably add some more calories to your eating plan when you're no longer trying to lose. But your basic eating habits will be the ones you established during your weight loss.

Have you forgotten that you promised yourself you'd focus on your health rather than on your appearance or the numbers on the scale? This would be a good time to engage in some serious self-talk. Make a list of all the ways you feel better as a result of the weight you've lost so far. This is also the time to look at all the ways you've succeeded in changing your eating and activity patterns. Pat yourself on the back for every time you've chosen vegetables over junk food and for every hour spent in the garden instead of in front of the TV. It all adds up. Give yourself a well-deserved reward that isn't food.

If your overall goals are too stringent, then you may need to reassess. For example, when Nancy (not her real name) decided to lose weight, she set her goal at 120 pounds, which was less than what she had weighed in high school. At 5'5", she thought that weight sounded nice and thin, almost Hollywood-thin. She lost the weight, but within 6 months gained it back, plus a few pounds. She realized that her goal had been unrealistic for her. The next time she decided to lose weight, she picked a realistic weight for her height and age and focused on her health. That time she was successful.

So if you're struggling, reassess your goals. Make sure they're your goals, not anyone else's, and make sure they're realistic.

A solution for every problem

You learned in Chapter 9 that there would be setbacks on your way to achieving a healthy weight and that it would be wise for you to have a plan for when you encountered those setbacks. When you find your progress blocked by a seemingly immovable object, it's time to dust off the old problem-solving skills and have at it.

The first thing you need to do is to clearly identify the problem. Maybe you eat according to your plan, making nutritious, low-fat food choices, until you go to a restaurant. There you throw caution to the winds. Like someone who's been stranded on an island without food for weeks, you devour the bread and butter the waiter puts on the table, order more food than you need or want, finish every bite and top it off with a rich dessert.

You know the problem. (There may be more than one problem for you to solve, but focus on one at a time.) The next step is to create a list of possible solutions. Use your imagination. Be creative. When your list is complete, evaluate the solutions you've listed. Then pick one and try it.

Maybe you lose control in restaurants because you feel deprived. You don't want to be nibbling on lettuce while others are enjoying their meals. So perhaps your solution is to order what you want, but eat only part of it. Ask the waiter to bring a to-go box as soon as you're satisfied but not stuffed, and put half or more of it away to eat at another time or to freeze.

You can also ask the waiter to have the chef make fat- and calorie-saving modifications to your meal. Order the Caesar salad, but ask for the dressing on the side and put on just enough for flavor. In a Chinese restaurant, request that a minimum of oil be used in stir-frying your dish. Have your omelet made with egg whites and half the cheese. Don't be shy. You're paying for the food. You should have it the way you want it. Won't you enjoy your meal more if you don't feel as though you're abandoning your healthy eating plan with every bite?

As for dessert, order one to share, or eat just a few bites and savor the heck out of each morsel. And remember, even if you don't eat out very often, this is not the last supper. You will eat again.

Whatever solution you pick, evaluate the success of it. If it worked, then you've got yourself a plan for eating in restaurants, or whatever your problem is. If it didn't work, try, try again. You already have alternatives on your list. Pick another solution and go through the same process until you find one that works for you.

Here are some common problems people face as they work to achieve their healthy weight and some possible solutions. Try these or see what others you can come up with. Be creative. You can even make a game out of it by having a brainstorming session with your support person or team.

Problem	Possible solution
No time to exercise	• Get up earlier and work out before work. • Work out on your lunch hour. • Work out in 2 or 3 10-minute sessions throughout the day. • Think activity rather than exercise. Mow the lawn, climb the stairs, park farther from your destination and walk more.
No time to prepare meals	• Try the quick, healthful recipes offered in this book and look for other such recipes. • Take advantage of salad bars and healthful fast food, such as veggie submarine sandwiches, pizza without cheese and deli sandwiches light on the meat and heavy on vegetables.
Late-night snacking	• Don't skip meals. Make sure you're eating enough during the day. • Don't bring snack foods into the house. • Take up an activity that keeps you busy or gets you out of the house.
Sampling while cooking	• Chew gum or suck on a mint. • Have cut-up vegetables on hand and munch on them. • Have someone else do taste-testing for you.

If you can't identify a particular problem that's blocking your progress, then perhaps you've lost your motivation. In that case, go back to weighing the pros and cons, as described in Chapter 9. List the benefits of staying with your lifestyle changes, then list all the things you dislike about your new behaviors. Say you love the way your yoga class makes you feel, but you hate the time it takes. If your cons outweigh your pros, then you need to focus on the pros and use your problem-solving skills to find solutions to the cons, just as you did initially. It's normal for your motivation to fluctuate, so it's not unusual to have to beef it up from time to time. That's all right. Just be prepared, and don't get discouraged.

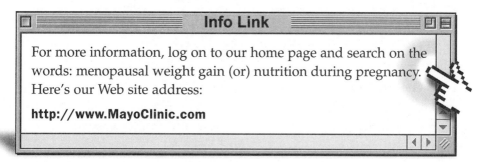

Info Link

For more information, log on to our home page and search on the words: menopausal weight gain (or) nutrition during pregnancy. Here's our Web site address:

http://www.MayoClinic.com

Willpower vs. self-control

To achieve any goal, you have to be flexible. That's why it's important not to get caught up in perfectionist, all-or-nothing thinking. Some people think they can achieve healthy weight if they just exert enough willpower. Perhaps you know yourself well enough to know that you can exert a lot of willpower for a long time. That is, after all, how you lost weight in the past. But what happens when your willpower cracks? You not only find yourself blowing your food plan for now, but you're likely to tell yourself you've failed, so why bother to try. That is, after all, how you gained weight back in the past.

Think about this: Say that before you started your new food and activity plan, you learned from your food diary you have a voracious sweet tooth. You can approach that problem in two ways. One is to ask yourself how you can fit occasional sweets into your program without destroying your overall plan. Two is to tell yourself you'll avoid sweets entirely. If you choose plan number two, then you have to exert a tremendous amount of willpower. Let's face it. If you like sweets, you're going to feel deprived when you can't have them. And deprivation, as we saw in Chapter 9, is likely to lead to binge eating.

So you tell yourself you can have some sweets in moderation. But you know you can never get enough Sara Lee cherry cheesecake. Here's the trick: Allow yourself to have some sweets. But instead of using your willpower to avoid cheesecake, use self-control.

What's the difference? Self-control is, "Cheesecake is my problem food, so I'm not going to keep it in the house." Willpower is, "I'm going to buy my favorite cheesecake, but I'm not going to eat it. I'll prove to myself how strong my willpower is." Get real. The first approach is sensible planning; the second is torture. And since the lifestyle changes you make are supposed to be both healthy and pleasurable, why would you choose to torture yourself?

There's a "Cathy" cartoon in which Cathy is complaining to a friend that no matter how determined she is to avoid eating a doughnut, she ends up eating one every day. "Why not just keep doughnuts out of your house?" asks the friend. "What?" says Cathy. "And let them think they're winning?"

No one wins when you rely on your willpower and it fails you, as it inevitably will. So do as Cathy's wise friend suggests, and keep the temptations as far away from you as possible.

Take heart. Chances are, as your taste buds adapt to your new style of eating, cheesecake or doughnuts or whatever your downfall is will loosen its grip on you and won't taste as good as it once did. Barring that, look for a recipe for a lower-fat, lower-sugar version of your favorite treat, and indulge in small portions on occasion. If necessary, keep your treats hidden in the back of the freezer or cut off a small piece for yourself and give the rest away so you won't be tempted. You may be surprised to discover that just knowing it's all right to allow yourself a treat now and then can make it easier to say no.

There are ways of breaking the chain of behavior that leads to your overeating. Let's take a closer look.

Chain of behavior

In *The LEARN Program for Weight Control*, authors Brownell and Wadden suggest examining the behavior chain that leads to your overeating and then breaking the chain into discrete parts. Examining the parts will lead to ideas for stopping the behavior and increasing your understanding of why you eat unintentionally. They use the example of a woman named Laura, who ate 10 cookies, felt guilty, and ate some more. Here's her chain:

- Buy cookies (the trouble starts).
- Leave cookies on the counter (where they're clearly visible and tempting).
- Be home on Saturday afternoon (her high-risk time and place for overeating).
- Be tired and bored.
- Get the urge to eat.
- Go to the kitchen.
- Take cookies to the den.
- Eat cookies while watching TV.
- Eat rapidly until full.
- Feel guilty and like a failure.
- Restraint weakens further.
- Eat more.

Chances are you can identify a similar chain for yourself. The good thing is there are many opportunities for breaking the chain. Think about your own chain for a moment. Think about the sequence of events that leads to your eating episodes. Now think about link-breaking techniques.

In Laura's case, she could have stopped herself from buying the cookies in the first place by shopping from a list, shopping on a full stomach, shopping with a partner who was aware of her temptations, or buying a cookie mix that needed baking. When she got home, she could have stored the cookies out of sight. She could have frozen them. Knowing Saturday afternoon was a high-risk time for out-of-control eating, she could have planned an activity that kept her occupied or took her away from home.

At every link in the chain, she could have done something to break the chain of events. You can do the same with your chain.

Brownell and Wadden suggest going after the weakest link and interrupting the chain as early as possible. For example, if ice cream lures you into overeating, then it might be better not to buy it or to buy a flavor you don't like rather than to trying to avoid eating it once it's in your freezer. Again, self-control is easier to exercise than willpower. Lead yourself not into temptation.

Friends in need

In Chapter 9, we talked about the importance of enlisting support in your healthy weight efforts. If you pooh-poohed that piece of advice, and you're now finding the going rough, then you might want to consider finding a coach, such as a dietitian or therapist, or joining a commercial group of like-minded people. Being with others who are experiencing similar challenges could be invaluable, especially if you haven't found support for your efforts elsewhere.

We all like to think we're pretty tough and that we can handle our lives ourselves. But you're going through some big, difficult changes here. Getting support for your efforts, whether through an individual who's a professional or from a group of fellow travelers on this path, could ultimately mean the difference between success and failure. Joining with people engaged in a similar struggle can give you just the boost you need to overcome the inevitable obstacles and setbacks you'll face along the way.

If you consider joining a commercial program, however, exercise caution. You want a program whose methods and goals are consistent with achieving and maintaining a healthy weight. You'll find programs listed in the Yellow Pages under "weight control services." Along with the ones worth considering, such as Take Off Pounds Sensibly (TOPS) and Weight Watchers, you'll find other organizations that make promises they can't and shouldn't keep.

If you do join a group, keep in mind that what you'll get out of it will be in proportion to what you put into it. If you sit in a corner and just listen, you may hear some good suggestions. But if you participate, you're more likely to reap the rewards of the group, which include support, encouragement, feeling that you're not alone, and suggestions specific to your concerns. To be a good group member, be willing to give as well as receive. Listen to others, contribute to the conversation, but don't monopolize it, don't judge, and be supportive.

Staying the course

You may think that once you've achieved a healthy weight, your work is done. Once you've reached your goal, staying there should be a breeze. Sorry, but that's your old diet mentality talking. It goes back to the idea that you go on a diet to lose weight, and once you lose, you go off. That kind of thinking leads to regaining weight. Been there, done that. Not going there again.

This time you're going to hold on to your hard-won victory. Maintaining weight involves the same process as losing it. You can probably add some calories to your daily intake once you reach your goal weight. Besides that, you just need to keep walking the path you're on. Whatever you employed to help you lose weight, you'll need to use to keep it off.

That's why we've been stressing the need for lifestyle changes. That's why it's so important to make changes you can live with over the long haul. You're already doing what you need to do. You're making healthy food choices and moving your body every day. You look good. You feel good. You're justifiably proud of yourself. Just keep on keeping on.

Defining success

Don't depend on your mirror when it comes to measuring the success of your efforts to achieve a healthy weight. Your mirror won't reveal the factors that really count. Are you feeling better? Are you eating better? Are you more active? Have you gained muscle? Have your blood pressure and blood fats improved? Have you lost inches as well as weight? Are you positioned to maintain the weight loss?

Twenty years of weight loss

I'm not sure how much I weighed at my peak. I avoided scales. But I'm sure I was 215 pounds or more — too heavy for my 5-foot 5-inch frame. I know I was a size 22.

That's history. For the past 20 years, I've weighed between 140 and 145 pounds. On March 1, 1979, I made a lifetime commitment to lose weight and keep it off. I didn't like how I felt. Though I was only 26 years old, I felt old. I felt limited in my activities. I felt like I couldn't wear what I wanted to wear.

I put on my sweat suit. It was tight, and I didn't feel confident about exercising. But I determined to run every day for a year. I never missed one of those 365 days. One thing I learned is you get kind of compulsive when you start something, and then you begin to balance out. Now I exercise 30 to 45 minutes, 5 or 6 days a week. I started with jogging, but as I became healthier, I added other activities: tennis, racquetball, ball, skiing, swimming. I run in one or two races a year partly because I like the T-shirts I get. They're a symbol of victory to me. I'm going to make them into a quilt someday.

Exercise is what helps me most, because it's a victory that's contagious. For me, victory in exercising leads to victory in diet. If I go through a hard time where I overeat, or if it's Christmas — when I choose to enjoy sweets — I can still exercise. And if my weight hits 152 or 153 — I prefer to measure with my tight jeans instead of scales — I start a food diary to get back on track.

Besides helping me keep tabs on what I eat, the food journal has helped me identify my vulnerable eating times. One of those times is what I called the 5 o'clock frenzy. Especially when my girls were younger, I'd rush home from work, hungry and worn out. I'd start cooking and eat while I cooked. But I learned that I could take the edge off being ravenously hungry by taking an apple or a bag of carrots to work, and then snacking on them during the drive home.

I don't eat perfectly. But I do make daily menus and shop from that list. And though I love sweets, and refuse to give them up entirely, I generally reserve them for an occasional treat on the weekends. One thing I've noticed is that sweets aren't what they used to be. I used to love doughnuts. But now I have maybe one a month. I've gradually seen a change in what I desire to eat. Still, I have setbacks. I may see brownies on the kitchen counter and eat more than I should. But then I say to myself that tomorrow's a new day. And I'm up at 5:30 the next morning to exercise.

As I get older, it's harder to keep the weight off. I added lifting weights about 3 to 4 years ago. I spend only about 15 minutes, three times a week. I do it mostly to maintain my weight loss, but I also need it for my osteoporosis prevention and because women lose their muscle mass big time as they grow older.

I have to be honest, every day takes a new commitment. I'm moving into another house right now, so I'm tired. But I know I need to do 30 to 45 minutes of my Nordic Track and treadmill, which is my main exercise during these Minnesota winters.

I look in the mirror and still can't believe what I see — even after 20 years. I still have the mental image that I'm overweight. Those kinds of memories stay in your head a long time. But the reality is the picture I see in the mirror, and the solid record of good health. I haven't needed to take a sick day in 18 years.

Faye
Byron, Minnesota

And finally . . .

You've heard the grim statistic about the likelihood of losing weight and keeping it off permanently — 95 percent who lose weight regain it within 5 years.

How discouraging. If you're experiencing a rough spot in your healthy weight efforts, then the last thing you need is bad news. So how about this: You are not doomed to failure. According to a study published in the *American Journal of Clinical Nutrition* of folks who participated in the National Weight Control Registry (NWCR), hundreds of people succeed at reaching and maintaining a healthy weight.

In fact, the study followed 629 women and 155 men who had been overweight for years. They lost an average of 66 pounds. And, yes, they did gain some back. But they kept a minimum of 30 pounds off for at least 5 years. Most of them did it through a combination of restricting fat and calories and exercising. They did it by making the very lifestyle changes we're recommending to you. A big surprise of the study was that 42 percent of the participants said that maintaining their healthy weight was easier than losing the weight in the first place.

The best news is that 95 percent of the people involved gave a big thumbs-up to their weight loss. They said it improved the quality of their lives, including their mood, their health and their self-confidence. In case you doubt it, they're here to tell you that life is better when you achieve a healthy weight.

So forget all those reports about weight-loss failures and how hard it is to maintain a healthy weight. The people of the NWCR are living testimony that it can be done and that it's worth doing. When the going gets tough, use your problem-solving skills, question the beliefs that underlie your habits, get the support you need, rely on self-control instead of willpower, and think of the folks of the NWCR.

They did it, and so can you.

Other eating plans

If achieving a healthy weight were completely easy, there wouldn't be so many weight-loss programs and products out there. In fact, Americans spend more than $34 billion a year on various diet aids and services, looking for the magic cure that will help them shed pounds quickly and painlessly. This year, nearly 51 million Americans will enroll in some kind of structured weight-reduction program.

Unfortunately, people often find that whatever pounds they drop come right back, in part because they get tired of avoiding bread or loading up on grapefruit or feeling hungry while existing on very few calories. Even worthy diet plans will fail when good intentions can't overcome a feeble commitment to making permanent lifestyle changes.

It's easy enough to lose weight quickly on any popular diet, in part because they all restrict calories. A calorie is a calorie, no matter where it comes from or how it's consumed, and when you eat fewer of them you're bound to lose weight. You can do this on your own — without the benefit of *The Zone* or *Sugar Busters* or the Beverly Hills Diet — simply with a more active lifestyle and by replacing the foods you obsess over with a lower-calorie diet based on the Mayo Clinic

Healthy Weight Pyramid.

Most people underestimate the number of calories they eat by at least 20 percent — more if they're very overweight. You may think you're holding your calorie level to 1,500 a day, for example, when you're really consuming closer to 1,800. People also misjudge their physical activity, believing a walk from the car to the office will suffice for half their day's needed exertion.

Some structured diet plans try to quantify what you eat, by requiring that you count fat grams or by allotting points to the foods you eat. Although these systems may not be the ultimate solution to your weight-loss quandary, they may help you see a more direct relationship between what you put in your mouth and its eventual effects on your body. Of course, you'll also want to make long-term changes that will result in a healthful, sustainable way of eating.

Here are some of the popular diets in circulation today.

Low-calorie liquid diets

There are two kinds of very-low-calorie liquid-based diets (VLCDs): those that are given under medical supervision, such as Medifast and Optifast, and those you can buy over the counter, such as Slim-Fast.

Medifast and Optifast usually are prescribed as an intervention for seriously overweight people for whom nothing else has worked. Not intended as a long-term solution — since these diets restrict calories to about 800 a day — Medifast and Optifast usually include an initial phase, followed by a moderate calorie-restricted diet, behavior modification or drugs.

When VLCDs first came out, early studies showed they often resulted in serious health complications, even death. But products now contain supplements that provide necessary protein, minerals and other nutrients, which make them generally safe. Long-term results, however, have been no better than with behavioral modification alone.

If you're on a VLCD, or if you're considering one, it's important to have ongoing medical monitoring with your health care providers.

Over-the-counter plans suggest that you replace one to two

meals with their product, then eat a healthy, balanced third meal that should be low in fat and calories. Slim-Fast also recommends plenty of snacking on healthy foods, such as fruits and vegetables, and 30 minutes of activity a day.

Low-calorie solid-food diets

Cut calories, lose weight. If only diet experts saw it that simply. Yet countless theories exist about what kinds of calories will pack on the pounds and those that won't even count, what categories of foods will optimize your body's performance, and those that will slow it down.

The Atkins diet

Robert Atkins, M.D., was a pioneering proponent of a high-protein/low-carbohydrate diet back in the 1970s when his *Dr. Atkins' Diet Revolution* hit the bookstores. His ideas went out of vogue with the low-fat craze in the '90s, but he's selling books again with his *Dr. Atkins' New Diet Revolution*.

Dr. Atkins believes that carbohydrates promote insulin production, which leads to weight gain and other health risks. The Atkins diet, therefore, limits carbohydrates to 20 to 40 grams a day initially. Most grains, beans, fruits, breads, pastas and vegetables are excluded except for salad vegetables and small amounts of a few others. He says you can eat as much meat, eggs, cheese, butter and cream as you want.

Without enough dietary carbohydrates, your body begins to burn its stored carbohydrates (glycogen) for energy — which releases a lot of water weight. Your body also starts burning some fat, but not as efficiently as exercise would. Burning fat without carbohydrate creates toxic byproducts called ketones that build up in your bloodstream. These will be processed through your kidneys before they're eliminated.

To be sure, ketones suppress appetite, as Dr. Atkins says, but they also cause fatigue and nausea. The long-term health effects of this diet are unknown and potentially risky.

Ask yourself ...

If you're considering a new weight-loss plan, measure it by the following statements to see how the program holds up. If one or more of these apply, it should send up a red flag.

- Promises of a quick fix
- Dire warnings from a single product or regimen
- Claims that sound too good to be true
- Simplistic conclusions drawn from a complex study
- Recommendations based on a single study
- Dramatic statements that are refuted by reputable scientific organizations
- Lists of "good" and "bad" foods
- Advice given to help sell a product
- Opinions based on studies published without peer review
- Recommendations from studies that ignore differences among individuals or groups

Based on information from the Food and Nutrition Science Alliance

The Zone

Compared to Dr. Atkins, Barry Sears, Ph.D., author of *The Zone*, is downright permissive when it comes to carbohydrates. Sears claims the key to successful weight loss is a diet in which every meal has a carbohydrate-to-protein ratio of 4 to 3. For overweight people he recommends a caloric ratio of 40 percent carbohydrate, 30 percent protein and 30 percent fat. With this ratio, says Sears, dieters experience less hunger, increased energy, peak physical performance, improved mental focus and decreased illness.

The Zone diet's thrust is to sustain a specific ratio of insulin and glucagon, important regulators of carbohydrate metabolism. Maintaining the right proportion of these hormones, according to Sears, contributes to the balancing of eicosanoids, which are hormonelike substances derived from polyunsaturated fatty acids. The best way to enter "the Zone," says Sears, is by preserving your eicosanoid balance.

However, there is little evidence that eicosanoids are primarily responsible for diseases or that disease risk can be manipulated through changing eicosanoids in the diet. People will lose weight if they follow the prescribed diet in the book because it's low in total calories and emphasizes fruits and vegetables. A typical Zone diet consists of fewer than 1,000 calories a day.

Sugar Busters

When you consider that Americans each consume nearly three pounds of sugar per week, the premise of *Sugar Busters! Cut Sugar to Trim Fat* may seem like one whose time has come. But the concept — which lumps in whole foods such as potatoes, corn and carrots with refined sugars found in cakes, candies and sodas — goes too far. Moreover, while authors H. Leighton Steward and their associates don't advocate the heavy fats of Dr. Atkins, the diet still promotes its fair share of rich foods.

Cutting back on sugar is only one aspect of healthy dietary changes. Without making any other nutritional alterations, and particularly when encouraging the intake of saturated fat and decreasing beneficial vegetables, this diet is unlikely to help you lose weight — or at least keep it off over the long term.

Of course, you can find many other low-calorie-food-based diets besides the ones just mentioned. You've probably seen other high-protein/low-carbohydrate diets such as *Protein Power* and *The Carbohydrate Addict's Diet* books, or the Scarsdale diet, among many others. Although their methods differ, results are comparable to the weight-loss plans above.

Fad diets

Many diet plans sound downright unbelievable. It's hard to believe anyone would spend much time, for instance, eating only pineapple, corn and salad one day and prunes, strawberries and baked potatoes the next. Still, many similar weight-loss plans cause people to hope that a new food combination or nutritional revelation will help them lose those extra pounds once and for all.

Are these diets safe? As with the high-protein/low-carbohydrate

Questions and answers about fad diets

Why are fad diets so popular? Fad diets promote quick and easy weight loss. People tend to be interested in quick, simple solutions to problems. If you follow the plan, you may lose the weight quickly and relatively easily, but you'll gain it back. That's what's wrong with fad diets. They do not offer a permanent, healthy solution to the problem of overweight.

What's the worst aspect of fad dieting? This approach to weight loss may not be healthy in the long run. Diets shouldn't go against what we know about biochemistry and physiology, and about improving long-term health. Many of these diets advise reducing carbohydrate intake and include very few, if any, fruits, vegetables and grains.

There's a great deal of evidence that increasing fruits, vegetables, and whole grains, is good for your health. Eating a wide variety of fruits, vegetables and grains regularly, combined with daily physical activity, will promote permanent weight loss while helping to prevent serious illnesses such as cancer and heart disease.

On a fad diet, even if you lose weight you may not improve your long-term health. Although more traditional recommendations for weight management may seem old, boring and difficult, they lead to improved health as well as permanent weight loss.

diets and liquid diets, you'll probably grow tired of them before they can do any real damage. But the potential for harm arises if you attempt any long-term commitment to these dietary disasters. Will you lose weight? If you're cutting calories, you'll probably drop pounds, but the chances are good you'll gain them back once you go off any unsustainable diet.

Here are a few of the more popular fad diets:

Grapefruit diet

Although there are many versions of this plan (one even erroneously calls itself the Mayo Clinic Diet; see page 103), all require you to eat half a grapefruit before every meal to reap the benefits of the fruit's so-called fat-burning enzymes. Calories typically are limited to fewer than 800 a day, although some versions require that you eat until you are full.

Grapefruit has no fat, is low in calories and sodium, and is packed with vitamin C. But the very low calories — and deficits in protein, fiber and several important vitamins and minerals — can make this diet dangerous.

Beverly Hills diet

This is a short-term, quick weight-loss plan. Proponents suggest following it for only a month at a time. It relies mainly on food combinations, such as eating fruit by itself, and never eating protein with carbohydrates so that each food can be properly digested instead of stored as body fat.

Initial weight loss can be rapid, but the Beverly Hills diet employs extremely limited meal guidelines and is not based on any scientific evidence. The plan is also dangerously low in protein and several crucial vitamins and minerals. Here's a red flag: Champagne, on this diet, is unlimited.

Blood-type diet

This diet provides a very detailed list of foods that you should eat or avoid, depending on your blood type. Based on the book *Eat Right 4 Your Type* by Peter D'Adamo, the premise is that each blood type has its own unique antigen marker that reacts in negative ways with certain foods. Also, according to the book, individuals have varying levels of stomach acidity and digestive enzymes, which seem to correlate with blood type.

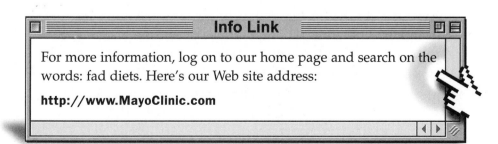

Info Link

For more information, log on to our home page and search on the words: fad diets. Here's our Web site address:

http://www.MayoClinic.com

Although you may find it comforting to have a list of foods to eat or avoid, there is no scientific evidence that diets should be based on blood type.

Cabbage soup diet

What could be simpler? Eat as much cabbage soup as you want for seven days and you'll lose 10 to 15 pounds. Other foods, too, are prescribed during the week long program, including potatoes, fruit juices and some vegetables.

The only problem is that cabbage soup proponents report feeling lightheaded and weak because the diet is too low in protein, vitamins and complex carbohydrates. You may lose weight, but you'll probably be too queasy to enjoy it.

Many, many other fad diets exist besides these few. If you were to try all of them, you'd be busy dieting and doing nothing else. Followers of the raw-foods diet, for example, consume only uncooked food; the Caveman diet allows you to eat only what Stone Age people ate; and *The Body Code,* by Jay Cooper, divides dieters into warriors, nurturers, communicators and visionaries.

Gwen Shamblin's *The Weigh Down Diet* advises using spirituality to avoid overeating; Harvey and Marilyn Diamond's *Fit for Life* recommends eating foods in specific combinations at certain times of the day; and Suzanne Somers' her books touting "Somercizing" involve very specific combinations of foods as well as the elimination of sugars and alcohol. You get the idea.

Prepared-food diets

Some people have a difficult time figuring out how they're supposed to eat in order to lose weight. In addition, busy schedules can preclude involved meal preparation or even keep you from trying new recipes. In those cases, calling on companies that will fix everything for you may deserve consideration. Remember, however, that these suppliers can be expensive. Some examples:

Jenny Craig

This plan started in 1983 by providing its clients with frozen meals. The company has since branched into cookbooks and programs that encourage clients to make food choices from readily available foods, as well as an at-home program for people who don't live close to an established center. Jenny Craig also encourages long-term weight loss through exercise, stress reduction and individual support.

Food is shipped to you overnight. You can receive personal consultations over the telephone. Using frozen meals is convenient, and the meals contain the right proportion of fat, carbohydrate, protein — all the necessary nutrients.

NutriSystem

NutriSystem also delivers frozen meals to your door for a set price per week. You select what you want for each meal, as well as seven desserts or snacks weekly. Meals are prepared in low-calorie portions that NutriSystem deems optimal for vitamins, minerals and other nutrients. You can choose from among NutriSystem's additional products, such as salad dressings, gelatins, crackers, rolls, beverages and skim milk alternatives.

Commercial group approaches

Even when you decide the best way to lose weight comes from eating low-calorie foods in moderate amounts and adding physical activity to your life, you don't have to go it alone. Commercial group programs can support your efforts, giving you eating plans, exercise recommendations and reinforcement from others on the same path.

Although some of these dietary approaches inspire camaraderie, they are different from fad diets in what they recommend. You won't find weird food combinations or burdensome consumption of any one item, for example. You won't be able to eat all the meat and cheese you want, but you won't grow sick at the sight of cabbage soup either.

Here's a sampling of group approaches that may help you make the kind of lifestyle changes that ultimately will reward you with a healthy weight you can maintain:

Weight Watchers

Since its founding in 1963, Weight Watchers has assisted millions of people worldwide in their quest to lose unwanted pounds. Today more than 1 million members gather each week at meetings around the world.

Weight Watchers believes in a healthful, comprehensive weight management program that includes plans for food, activity and behavior modification. Once you join, you attend a weekly

---

To join or not to join

How can you decide if a diet plan is right for you? A responsible and safe weight-loss program should include these five attributes:

1. **Safety.** Although a weight-management plan may be low in calories, it should include all of the recommended daily allowances (RDAs) for vitamins, minerals and protein.

2. **Slow and steady change.** You should lose weight at a gradual, yet steady, pace, unless your doctor believes you would benefit from a more rapid weight loss. With many calorie-restricted diets, you may lose quickly during the first week or two, but you should expect to lose 1 to 2 pounds a week after that.

3. **Doctor participation.** If you plan to lose more than 15 or 20 pounds, have any health problems or regularly take medication, see your doctor. Your physician will also know whether the weight-loss program you have in mind is appropriate, and how much weight you can sensibly lose.

4. **Help in changing your lifestyle.** Your weight-loss program should teach you how to permanently change your dietary habits and level of physical activity. Losing weight will be meaningless if you can't keep it off.

5. **Up-front information on fees.** You should know exactly how much the program will cost, with a detailed statement of fees and any expenses for additional items, such as dietary supplements.

meeting for a weigh-in, information or activity session and supportive conversation.

The program involves a 3-step approach encompassing the foods you eat, your activity levels and the use of specific strategies that promote long-term healthy weight. There's no measuring, no complicated counting, no forbidden foods.

The initial focus is on a 10 percent reduction in your weight. Once you reach that goal, you receive instruction and encouragement for continued weight loss. Eventually you reach your proper, healthy weight, and the focus moves to maintenance.

TOPS Club, Inc. (Take Off Pounds Sensibly)

This group was launched in 1948 and now has 275,000 members in 11,000 chapters in the United States and 20 foreign countries. Mainly a support group, TOPS doesn't tell you what foods to eat or how much to consume, nor does it watch over your exercise levels. It's a nonprofit, noncommercial group that's run solely by volunteers.

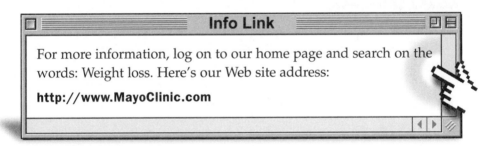

Info Link

For more information, log on to our home page and search on the words: Weight loss. Here's our Web site address:

http://www.MayoClinic.com

Weekly meetings begin with a confidential weigh-in, then include a program from a TOPS leader or member, or perhaps a physician, nutritionist, psychologist or other expert. Participants can share their successes and challenges in sessions afterward.

Before getting started, TOPS urges you to see your doctor for food and exercise plans, as well as an appropriate goal weight. The group does recommend an exchange dietary plan and publishes a healthy lifestyle guide that includes a full description of how to use the plan. Annual membership includes a monthly magazine delivered to your home.

Overeaters Anonymous

Are you a compulsive overeater? According to Overeaters Anonymous (OA), you're in the best position to decide whether your eating is out of control. If food has become unmanageable for you, Overeaters Anonymous can help. This is a program designed for people who regard themselves as recovering compulsive overeaters. The approach is identical to that of Alcoholics Anonymous, with 12 steps and 12 traditions. It's goal is to help members avoid compulsive overeating and to offer assistance to others who "still suffer."

OA takes no position on issues unrelated to overeating. It is not affiliated with private or public groups, ideologies or doctrines. The group is self-supporting, relying on contributions from members — there are no fees or dues. Donations are neither solicited nor accepted from non members.

Now's the time

If you have an eating disorder (see page 35), or if you're clinically depressed, treatment from a licensed mental health professional may be beneficial. Ask your physician for a referral. Some of these professionals specialize in treating people with weight or eating problems.

No matter what route you take on your trip toward healthy weight, it's important to get started now. Determine the eating plan that will work for you over the long haul, decide on an activity you can stick with, and identify the support system that will help you keep going even when the going gets tough.

The benefits of living at your healthy weight are numerous. You'll look better. You'll feel better. And you'll probably live longer, too. You don't have to go on a weight loss diet. You do have to change your life.

Part 3

When you need more help

Chapter 12
Medications for
weight loss   175
- Who's a candidate?   176
- Popular prescription
  medications   178
- Popular over-the-
  counter drugs   180
- Do you need a
  vitamin supplement?   183

Chapter 13
Surgery for weight loss   185
- Is surgery right for you?   186
- How your digestive
  system works   187
- Options to consider   188
- Side effects of surgery   192
- Making the adjustments 193
- It takes more than
  surgery   194

Appendix
Recipes you can rely on   195
- Sunshine juice blend   196
- Provencal chicken
  and fennel   196
- Summer savory spinach
  frittata   197
- Wild rice-and-chicken
  salad   198
- Thai-style mushroom-
  and-tofu stir-fry   199
- Gingered carrot soup   199

Chapter 12

Medications for weight loss

Take-home messages

- Diet and physical activity are the keys to healthy weight loss, even with weight-loss medications.
- Some medications are not effective for weight loss and should not be used.
- Medications have risks as well as potential benefits.
- See your physician or registered dietitian before taking a medication.

The newest medications for weight loss sound like a dieter's dream. One makes you feel full before you've eaten much. Another blocks your body's ability to absorb nearly a third of the fat you eat. But medications for weight loss aren't for everyone who's overweight. In fact, at Mayo Clinic they're generally reserved for people with weight-related health problems, such as high blood pressure, high cholesterol or diabetes.

It's best to lose weight through a healthy diet and regular exercise. Some people, however, have physical limitations that keep them from exercising. Others need extra help reducing their calorie intake. If you're among those who can't seem to lose weight on their own and the excess weight has produced medical problems — which can be improved or even eliminated by losing weight — medications may be able to help you.

Typically, the most popular prescription medications — combined with fewer calories and more activity — can help you lose anywhere from 5 percent to 10 percent of your total body weight within a year. The maximum weight loss usually peaks after about

6 months. However, many people gain back some of that weight in the second year. Also, the effectiveness and safety of the most popular prescription drugs haven't been tested beyond 2 years. It's the changes in diet and activity that will ultimately decrease weight and improve health. Drugs should be looked at as a tool to help make changes in diet, not as the answer to the problem.

Who's a candidate?

Doctors stress that medication for weight loss isn't meant for casual use, to lose a few pounds. Instead, these drugs are appropriate for moderately overweight and obese people who have health complications related to weight and who are enrolled in a weight-management program that emphasizes healthy nutrition and physical activity.

The main goal in using weight-loss medication is to improve your health, not your appearance. There are risks with each drug used, and doctors want to make sure the potential benefits out-weigh the risks.

If you're among the several million overweight Americans with medical complications, even a modest weight loss can improve your health in many ways, including lowering your blood pressure, your cholesterol, and your blood sugar level if you have diabetes.

There is no compelling evidence to suggest that using weight-loss drugs on otherwise healthy overweight people will prevent weight-related complications, improve the long-term outcome, or even lead to weight loss for more than 2 years.

If you're among those who can benefit from weight-loss medication, you'll likely need to take it indefinitely. Many studies show that when drug treatment is stopped, much or all of the excess weight generally returns. The dilemma with taking the drugs indefinitely is that the most commonly used prescription drugs are so new that their long-term effects are unknown.

In general, doctors consider you a candidate for medication treatment only if your body mass index (BMI) is greater than 27 and other medical complications of obesity are present. Exactly

A drug no longer used

Until the fall of 1997, one of the most popular prescriptions for weight loss was a combination of appetite suppressants known as fen-phen (fenfluramine and phentermine). In the year earlier, doctors in the United States wrote 18 million prescriptions for fen-phen.

This combination of medications suppressed the appetite and helped many people lose weight. But in July 1997, Mayo Clinic and MeritCare, a clinic based in Fargo, N.D., broke the news that some people taking these combined drugs were having unusual heart valve problems.

In their study, 24 women who were taking the drug combination and had no known history of heart disease all had heart valve trouble. Five required surgery. The valves became thick and covered with white plaque. As a result, the damaged valves allowed blood pumped through the valves to leak back in, forcing the heart to work harder. Later, data provided by the Food and Drug Administration (FDA) showed that up to 30 percent of the users of this combination might have heart valve abnormalities, even though they didn't have symptoms.

Based on this information, and at the request of the FDA, the manufacturers of fenfluramine and dexfenfluramine voluntarily withdrew these medications from the market in September 1997. Evidence suggested that fenfluramine, not phentermine, was the source of the problem. No direct evidence pointed to phentermine, which is still available by prescription. Phentermine was originally approved for only a 3-month use. Its long-term safety and effectiveness haven't been carefully studied.

Later studies suggested that heart valve disease affects about 1 in 4 who take the drugs. A study at Mayo Clinic reported that the damage may not be permanent — at least in people with mild disease. For these people, the abnormalities improve or disappear over time after discontinuing the drugs. If you took fenfluramine or dexfenfluramine, see your doctor to discuss further recommendations.

how many pounds overweight that is depends on your height, since your BMI is calculated from the ratio of your weight to your height. (See page 16.) But for people of average height (about 5 feet 10 inches for men and 5 feet 6 inches for women), it's roughly 20-30 pounds overweight.

Even if you qualify for weight-loss drug therapy, the drugs might not work for you. Studies suggest that if you don't lose at least 4 pounds within the first month on a particular medication, it's probably not going to help you. In that case, your doctor will likely take you off the drug and perhaps try another.

Popular prescription medications

Doctors today generally prescribe one of two drugs for weight loss. These drugs work in different ways and have different side effects. But in general, both appear generally safe and moderately effective for at least a year or two. Studies are under way to determine the safety and effectiveness beyond this length of time.

The 'I feel full' drug

The first weight-loss drug approved by the FDA after the popular drugs fenfluramine and dexfenfluramine were withdrawn from the market in 1997 was Meridia (sibutramine). Though this new drug doesn't seem to decrease your appetite, it changes your brain chemistry — mainly affecting serotonin and norepinephrine — making you feel full more quickly.

You generally take Meridia once a day with a full glass of water, with or without food. The recommended dose is 10 milligrams, though your doctor may have you take 5 milligrams if 10 milligrams is too much for you to tolerate, or 15 milligrams if the 10 milligram dose doesn't work. Though Meridia is convenient to take and generally does help you lose more weight than you could through diet and exercise alone, it's no magic bullet. In a 1-year study, Meridia users lost an average of 7 to 10 pounds more than people simply following a low-calorie diet and taking a placebo. However, this additional amount of weight loss may improve control of some health conditions associated with obesity, such as diabetes.

Meridia isn't without risks. It can cause a small increase in blood pressure. For some people, the increase can be high enough to warrant discontinuing the drug. Because of this, Meridia isn't recommended for people with uncontrolled high blood pressure, heart disease, irregular heartbeat or a history of stroke. And if you do take Meridia, the FDA recommends that you carefully monitor your blood pressure. Also, you shouldn't take the drug if you're pregnant or breast-feeding, because it's still uncertain whether the drug can harm your child.

The most common side effects noticed during treatment with Meridia are headache, dry mouth, constipation and insomnia.

The fat-blocker

In April 1999, the FDA approved a drug called Xenical (orlistat), the first in a new class of weight-loss medications. Unlike other drugs, which work through your central nervous system, Xenical acts only in your digestive tract, then passes out of your body, unabsorbed.

Xenical blocks natural enzymes needed to digest fat in the foods you eat. So just as indigestible fiber in grains and vegetables passes completely through your digestive system, so does about 30 percent of the fat you eat when you take Xenical. The recommended dose is 120 milligrams up to three times a day, with meals that contain fat.

Average weight loss, however, is modest — and similar to what you could expect with Meridia. In clinical trials, most people on reduced-calorie diets who took Xenical for a year lost between 5 percent and 10 percent of their initial weight. In a 1-year study of people on a low-calorie diet, those taking Xenical lost an average of 22 pounds. Those taking a placebo lost 13 pounds. Studies lasting up to 2 years, however, show that a fourth to a third of the weight lost in the first year is generally regained in the second year. Still, the overall weight loss is often enough to improve your health.

Because the drug isn't absorbed by your body, you avoid potentially serious side effects such as heart valve disease. The side effects that you do experience are usually limited to your digestive system and are often only temporary:

- Oily rectal seepage or spotting
- Passing gas with discharge
- Sudden bowel movements, creating a sense of urgency
- Fatty or oily stools

These problems affect about 1 in 5 people taking Xenical, but the symptoms are generally mild. The more fat you eat, the more symptoms you have. Studies show that by the second year, and most often much sooner, symptoms have disappeared. In a way, the symptoms might have some added benefit because they may discourage you from eating fatty foods.

Since Xenical blocks absorption of some nutrients, your doctor may recommend that you also take a multivitamin containing the fat-soluble vitamins A, D, E and K. This should be taken 2 hours before or 2 hours after Xenical.

Popular over-the-counter drugs

Over-the-counter (OTC) diet products are a huge success — for the companies that manufacture them. Sales have climbed steadily, creating an almost $6 billion industry. Unfortunately, you can't count on these diet aids to lighten anything but your wallet. And worse, some OTC diet drugs can do far more harm than good.

Most of these weight-loss products promise to help you shed pounds by raising your metabolism or suppressing your appetite. The side effects, however, can be dangerous. And the lost weight is almost always temporary.

Here's a look at some of the more popular OTC diet medications and what they will and won't do for you.

Ephedrine
One of the most popular OTC weight-loss products is Metabolife, an herbal dietary supplement that earned $600 million in sales in 1998. Similar products are Metab-O-LITE and MetaboMax, but the main ingredient in all of these is ephedrine, which comes from the ephedra plant or can be made synthetically.

Ephedrine has long been used in asthma medicine, but it's also used to make the street drug methamphetamine, commonly known as speed. Chemically, there's only a slight difference between methamphetamine and ephedrine.

This drug can slightly suppress your appetite. It can also cause high blood pressure, heart rate irregularities, insomnia, nervousness, tremors, seizures, heart attacks, strokes and death.

Although the FDA has received hundreds of reports of adverse effects from ephedrine, including deaths, herbal diet supplements aren't classified as drugs, so the FDA has no power to approve or ban them, as it does with drugs. For safety's sake, the FDA has proposed limiting ephedrine to less than 8 milligrams per serving of a product and limiting its use to no more than 7 days, which renders it useless as a diet aid.

Even if Metabolife or other products containing ephedrine were to help you lose weight, you'd have to continue taking the product to keep the weight off. The short-term safety of ephedrine is questionable for this purpose, and the long-term effects are unknown.

Chitosan

This is a dietary supplement made from chitin, a starch found in the skeleton of shrimp, crab and other shellfish. Because chitosan (KITE-o-san) isn't digested, it passes through your intestinal tract unabsorbed, so it adds no calories. The chemical nature of chitosan makes it bind with fatty foods you eat, removing some of this fat from your body rather than allowing it to be absorbed. One study, however, found no more weight loss from chitosan than from a placebo.

Hydroxycitric acid

A common ingredient in herbal weight-loss products, hydroxycitric acid (HCA), comes from a plant native to India: *Garcinia cambogia.* Popular brand names of this herb include Citrus Slim Gum, CitriMax and CitraLean. A study in the *Journal of the American Medical Association* in 1998 found the herb ineffective for weight loss. In this study, people taking HCA and eating a low-calorie diet lost no more weight than people on the same diet and taking a placebo. In fact, the people on the placebo lost slightly more weight.

Saint John's wort

This is an herbal medicine derived from the *Hypericum perforatum* plant. European studies suggest it may work for relieving depression. But the FDA says this herbal medication hasn't been proven safe or effective for weight loss, and it can interact with some prescription medications.

5-hydroxy-L-tryptophan (5-HTP)

Sold under brand names such as Natrol, Natural Balance, and Solaray, this extract from a plant seed contains a contaminant linked to a rare and potentially deadly blood disorder. Chemically, 5-HTP is closely related to L-tryptophan, a dietary supplement banned in 1990 after researchers found the same contaminant that has since been discovered in 5-HTP.

Herbal laxatives and diuretics

They cause you to lose water, and thus weight, but not fat. They can lower your potassium levels, causing heart and muscle problems. Also, if you use laxatives too often, your bowels start depending on them.

Caffeine

A few studies indicate that in people who exercise and eat a low-fat diet, consuming large amounts of caffeine or other stimulants may slightly enhance weight loss. But taken in large doses, caffeine can cause jitters, irritability, insomnia and high blood pressure. And if combined with other stimulants, such as ephedrine, the side effects may be more serious.

Appetite suppressants

Appetite suppressants, such as Dexatrim and Acutrim, contain phenylpropanolamine hydrochloride, a stimulant used in cough and cold medicines. These drugs are probably safe unless you have high blood pressure or heart problems, but you still have to control your appetite once you stop taking them. Otherwise, you'll gain back the small amount of weight you lost, if any.

Pyruvate

This popular weight-loss dietary supplement may have a slight effect in helping you shed pounds, according to studies in the *American Journal of Clinical Nutrition*. Pyruvate, in the form of pyruvic acid, is found in various places. It is formed in the body during digestion of carbohydrates and protein. It's also in several foods, such as red apples, cheese and red wine. Pyruvate seems safe, but its claims of boosting metabolism, decreasing appetite, and weight loss need further study.

A word to the wise

People tend to take OTC drugs and herbs less seriously than prescriptions, and often take too much or mix them with other drugs. Also, because the manufacturing of herbs is unregulated by the FDA, you can't be sure what you're getting.

If you're troubled by your weight or have a medical condition that's worsened by your extra pounds, talk to your doctor. Whether you have 5 or 100 pounds to lose, you have to eat right and exercise to control your weight. OTC diet drugs can't help you with anything beyond short-term, temporary weight loss — if that. These diet products are more harmful than helpful.

Do you need a vitamin supplement?

The best way to get the vitamins and minerals you need is through a nutritionally balanced diet. A vitamin supplement may be appropriate if:

- **You're on a very-low-calorie diet.** If you eat fewer than 1,000 calories daily, you may need a supplement. Remember: A very-low-calorie diet limits the types and amounts of foods you eat and, in turn, the types and amounts of nutrients you receive. Don't go on a very-low-calorie diet without assistance from a physician.
- **You're on a special diet.** If your diet has limited variety because of intolerance or food allergy, you may need a supplement. If you're a vegetarian who eliminates all animal

products from your diet, you may need additional vitamin B-12. Also, if you don't eat dairy products and don't get 15 minutes of sun on your hands and face daily, you may need to supplement your diet with calcium and vitamin D.

- **You're 65 or older.** As you age, health problems can contribute to a poor diet, making it difficult for you to get the vitamins and minerals you need. You may lose your appetite. Your ability to taste and smell food may be diminished. Depression or problems with dentures can also inhibit eating. Also, your body may be unable to absorb vitamins B-6, B-12 and D as it used to.

- **You no longer have menstrual periods.** At menopause, it can be difficult for a woman to get the recommended amounts of calcium and vitamin D without supplementation. Calcium and vitamin D can help prevent osteoporosis.

- **You don't eat well.** If you eat alone you may not eat enough of the right kinds of foods.

- **You smoke or chew tobacco.** The use of tobacco products decreases the level of vitamins (especially vitamin C) and other nutrients in your blood and tissues.

- **You drink alcohol excessively.** Alcohol can impair digestion and absorption of thiamin, folate and vitamins A, D and B-12. Excessive drinking is more than one drink a day if you're a nonpregnant woman, and more than two a day if you're a man.

- **You're pregnant or breast-feeding.** You need more folic acid and iron if you're pregnant or breast-feeding. Begin the supplements before you become pregnant.

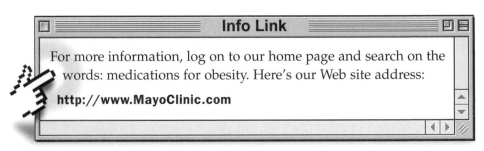

Info Link

For more information, log on to our home page and search on the words: medications for obesity. Here's our Web site address:

http://www.MayoClinic.com

Chapter 13

Surgery for weight loss

- If you are severely obese and nothing else has helped you lose weight . . .
- If you have medical problems that weight loss may help resolve . . .
- If you're willing to deal with substantial lifestyle changes . . .
- If you clearly understand the risks . . .
- Then, consider surgery for weight loss.

Surgery is no easy fix for your weight problem, but sometimes it can accomplish what exercise and a healthy diet alone can't. Surgery for weight loss is generally reserved for people who are severely overweight and who have health problems as a result.

The most common weight-loss surgery does two things. First, it blocks off part of your stomach, limiting how much you can comfortably eat. Second, it tends to prevent you from eating high-calorie sweets because of a side effect known as the dumping syndrome. Drinking soda pop on an empty stomach, for example, can result in the liquid moving too quickly through your digestive system, causing nausea, sweating and shakiness — symptoms of the dumping syndrome.

Surgery alone won't solve your weight problem. But if you're committed to losing weight and if the surgery is accompanied by a healthy diet, exercise and a positive outlook, you have an excellent chance of losing much of your excess weight — and then keeping it off. One study reports that 3 years after surgery, nearly 3 of every 4 patients had lost at least half their excess weight.

Is surgery right for you?

If you've tried to lose weight but remain severely obese and have weight-related health problems, surgery may be the next best step.

But first, you'll want to make sure you've made every effort to exercise and to change your eating habits and any lifestyle situations that have contributed to your weight gain. Surgery is not a replacement for these. In fact, the success of your surgery will depend at least partly on your commitment to carefully following the guidelines given to you about food choices and exercise.

For these reasons, candidates for surgery meet with health care workers from several disciplines. A physician nutritionist will evaluate your need for surgery, explain how the surgery will change the way your body receives and handles the nutrients it needs, and will discuss with you the importance of carefully following nutritional guidelines you'll receive. Your physician will also arrange a long-term monitoring program you'll need to follow after surgery. A dietitian will help you make healthful food selections before and after surgery. A psychologist will discuss social and psychologic problems you may face, as well as help you make lifestyle changes that encourage exercise and healthy eating.

A surgeon will evaluate you as a surgical candidate. If you're a candidate, the surgery will be scheduled. Even after your surgery, you'll continue to meet with health care professionals at least every 3 months for the first year, and then at least annually, so they can help you make the necessary changes in your life.

You may be a candidate for surgery if you fall into both of the following two categories:

Body mass index above 40

Your doctor may consider surgery if your body mass index (BMI, see page 16) is above 40, an indication that you are severely obese. Exactly how much overweight this is depends on the ratio between your weight and height. A man of average height generally reaches a BMI of 40 when he weighs 280 pounds.

For women, it's about 240 pounds. (To calculate your BMI, see page 16.)

Weight-related health problems
Doctors at Mayo Clinic generally won't perform the surgery simply because you have a BMI above 40, unless you are at high risk of certain health problems based on your lifestyle or family medical history. You need also have a weight-related health problem that will likely improve once you lose weight. Excessive weight can produce many medical problems, including high blood pressure, heart disease, diabetes, degenerative joint disease, and obstructive sleep apnea, which causes you to temporarily but repeatedly stop breathing at night, rousing you from a deep sleep and leaving you tired during the day.

In some cases, Mayo doctors will perform surgery if your BMI is as low as 35, if your related health problems warrant it. Some health care centers will perform surgery even if you have no weight-related health problems — as long as your BMI is above 40 — because of potential health problems that might be avoided with surgery.

How your digestive system works

Once you understand how your digestive system works, it's easier to see how surgery can help reduce weight. After you chew and swallow your food, muscles in your esophagus propel it into your stomach, which can hold about a quart and a half of food at one time. Digestive juices and the churning action of your stomach muscles break down the food into a mostly liquid mixture.

The stomach contents are then gradually released through a small opening (the pyloric valve) into your small intestine, which is about 18 feet long. Here is where most of the food nutrients are absorbed into your bloodstream.

After the food residue passes through your small intestine, it enters your large intestine — your colon — which eliminates undigested and unabsorbed particles and other waste products from your body.

Options to consider

Since the 1950s, when surgery for obesity began, doctors have used various operations to produce weight loss. Today, the most common operations fall into one of two categories.

The first uses a band or staples to create a small pouch at the top of your stomach, where food enters from your esophagus. The pouch can hold only about an ounce or two of food, though this can later expand to several ounces. After the operation, you can eat only small portions of food at a time without feeling nausea or discomfort.

The second type of surgery also creates a small pouch, but adds a bypass around part of your small intestine. This surgery does double duty. It reduces what you can eat, and it reduces the calories your body absorbs.

Here are some of the specific operations, representing these two categories:

Small-bowel bypass

This is an example of the second category of surgery. Also called a jejunoileal bypass, this was the first operation for obesity. This surgery takes your food on a bypass from your stomach to your colon, skipping almost all of your small intestine. As a result, most of the food you eat never comes in contact with the absorptive area of your intestine, so nearly all the nutrition is lost.

People lose a large amount of weight with this surgery, but many also experience severe complications: liver failure, arthritis, kidney stones and severe

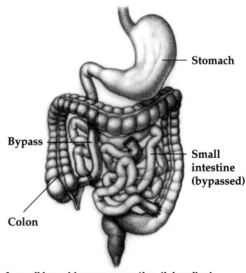

A small-bowel bypass operation (jejunoileal bypass) takes your food on a bypass from your stomach directly to your colon. If you've had this outdated procedure and you seem to have serious medical problems related to this operation, see your physician about having it reversed.

diarrhea. For this reason, this operation is no longer performed. Many doctors recommend that people who underwent this operation have it reversed if they have active complications.

Gastric partitioning

Also known as gastric stapling, this is an operation that divides your stomach into a tiny upper pouch and a large lower pouch.

In one technique, the surgeon uses a surgical stapler to apply a horizontal row of staples, dividing your stomach into two sections. The surgeon leaves a dime-sized opening between the two sections. Although this is a faster and slightly safer procedure than some more common operations, the weight loss has been disappointing. This is probably because the opening between the two stomach pouches gradually dilates and grows bigger, therefore defeating the purpose of the operation. Most surgeons no longer perform this surgery.

Another technique, especially popular in Europe, is called gastric banding. The surgeon uses a band instead of staples to partition the stomach into two parts. This band is wrapped around the upper part of your stomach and pulled tight, like a belt, creating a tiny channel between the two pouches. The band helps protect the opening from expanding. Surgeons are able to perform this procedure with tiny incisions through a laparoscope, a tube through which they can insert slender instruments. A tiny camera on the tip of the scope allows the surgeons to see inside you. Many doctors in the United States have reservations

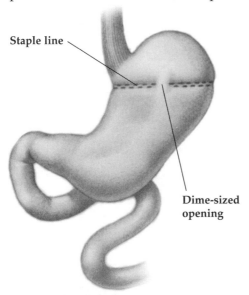

Staple line

Dime-sized opening

Gastric partitioning (gastric stapling) horizontally divides your stomach into a tiny upper and a larger lower pouch, and leaves a small opening between the two.

about the long-term effects of this surgery, and don't currently perform the procedure. It is considered experimental.

Vertical-banded gastroplasty

Called VBG for short, this is an example of the first category of surgery, which is designed to partition the stomach into two parts. There is no bypass. Using a surgical stapler, the surgeon divides your stomach into upper and lower sections. The upper pouch is small and empties into the lower pouch, which is the rest of your stomach.

At the dime-sized opening where the upper pouch empties into the rest of your stomach, the surgeon wraps the tissue with a piece of nonexpandable plastic. This "banding" of the opening between the upper stomach pouch and the rest of the stomach helps prevent the opening from stretching. If the opening stretches enough, the two pouches essentially become one again, defeating the purpose of the surgery.

This surgical procedure is called a vertical-banded gastroplasty because the staple line creating the upper pouch is placed vertically (up and down) on the stomach and the opening of the upper pouch is banded. About 3 in 10 people who have this surgery eventually lose about half of their excess weight. About 7 in 10 experience at least some weight loss, but many fail to maintain the weight loss initially achieved. They may adapt to eating smaller amounts of food at a time, but continue eating unhealthful foods and failing to exercise. Also, this operation works by limiting the amount of "meat and

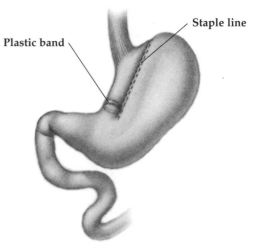

Plastic band · Staple line

A vertical-banded gastroplasty divides your stomach into upper and lower sections. The upper pouch holds only 1 ounce of food, so you feel full sooner. Food is released into the lower section through a small opening reinforced by a plastic band that helps prevent expansion of the opening.

potatoes" you're able to eat. But ice cream, milkshakes and other high-calorie liquids or soft sweets can slide through the opening with little resistance. Surgery alone isn't enough.

The main complication of this surgery is narrowing of the banded opening. It happens in about 1 in 50 cases. This reduces the food's ability to leave the upper pouch, which causes repeated vomiting and, often, heartburn. Another operation may be required to correct the problem. This can usually be done in an outpatient procedure that expands the opening with a dilating tube inserted into your stomach through your mouth.

Gastric bypass

This is the weight-loss surgery most often recommended by doctors. It's the second type of operation mentioned earlier — one using a small pouch, but adding a bypass around part of your small intestine.

The surgeon staples your stomach all the way across the top, leaving a tiny pouch that holds about half an ounce. Then the surgeon cuts the small intestine and sews a part of it directly onto the upper pouch. This redirects the food, bypassing most of your stomach and the first section of your small intestine, the duodenum (do-oh-DEE-num). Food flows directly into the middle section of your small intestine, the jejunum (juh-JOO-num), limiting your body's ability to absorb calories.

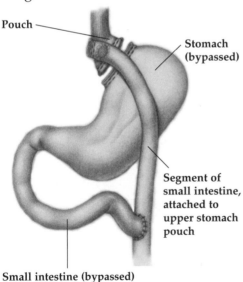

Pouch

Stomach (bypassed)

Segment of small intestine, attached to upper stomach pouch

Small intestine (bypassed)

Gastric bypass creates a small pouch at the top of your stomach and a bypass around most of your stomach and part of your small intestine. Most surgeons prefer this procedure.

Even though food never enters the lower part of your stomach, the stomach stays healthy and continues making digestive juices that flow into your small intestine.

Most surgeons prefer this

procedure because it has been proved safe and has few complications. Also, research shows that weight loss is encouraging and usually maintained. Most people lose at least half their excess weight.

As a rare but possible side effect, the opening between your stomach and small intestine can narrow. This may require corrective surgery or, more commonly, an outpatient procedure that stretches the opening with a dilating tube passed through your mouth.

Other more common but less serious side effects include deficiency of iron, which is needed to make red blood cells, and vitamin B-12, needed to make white blood cells and to allow nerves to work normally. All people undergoing gastric bypass should take a daily multivitamin with iron, take calcium supplements and receive monthly injections of vitamin B-12 for the rest of their lives. Iron deficiency is usually a potential problem only in menstruating women, and can be reversed by taking pills that contain iron.

Other potential complications of this surgery include the dumping syndrome (see page 185) and a bleeding sore, or ulcer, that might develop where your small intestine is attached to the upper part of your stomach. This used to be a serious problem. It now occurs in only about 1 in 100 patients. The ulcer can often be healed with medicine, though corrective surgery might be needed.

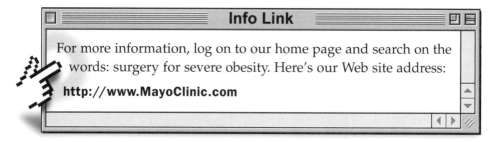

Info Link

For more information, log on to our home page and search on the words: surgery for severe obesity. Here's our Web site address:
http://www.MayoClinic.com

Side effects of surgery

No matter what kind of surgery you have, as you lose weight in the first months you may experience one or more of the following changes as your body reacts to the acute weight loss:

- Feeling tired, as if you have the flu

- Feeling cold, even when others feel comfortable
- Dry skin
- Hair loss (temporary)

These side effects usually go away in time.

A hernia or weakness may also develop at the site of your incision. This happens in about 15 percent of the people who have weight-loss surgery. A hernia will usually require surgical repair in the future, depending on the symptoms and the extent of the weakness.

Another side effect is that the faster you lose weight, the more muscle and lean tissue you lose along with fat. This is one reason it's important for you to exercise while losing weight. The exercise helps build your muscles while you lose fat tissue.

Making the adjustments

Many people underestimate the physical and social adjustments they'll have to make after surgery. You'll have a stomach about the size of a small egg. In the first 6 months after surgery, if you eat too much or too fast, you'll either get an intense pain under your breastbone that lasts for about 30 minutes or you'll vomit. Instead of eating regular-size meals three times a day, you'll be required to eat 4 to 6 meals (each about 2 ounces) throughout the day. Most people quickly learn how much they can eat at one time. With time, the amount you can eat (slowly) at one sitting will increase. By 1 year after the operation, you probably will be able to eat a half to three-fourths of a full sandwich, provided you eat it slowly and over a span of 45 minutes.

Dinner parties and eating out can be especially difficult to adjust to, at first. Everyone else is eating a regular meal, when all you're able to eat is a few bites.

The change in your body image may require other adjustments. Your new appearance can affect your relationships with friends, family and even your spouse, producing tension, anxiety and depression. This is one of the reasons you'll be asked to see a psychologist during an evaluation for your surgery.

It takes more than surgery

Surgery for weight reduction is not a miracle procedure. Though you can expect to lose weight and keep it off, especially if you have a gastric bypass, the changes needed in your eating and exercise habits are yours to make. But the pride and feeling of accomplishment as you lose weight, as well as the awareness of improved health, will be yours as well.

Liposuction: Not a weight-loss plan

Liposuction is cosmetic surgery, not a weight-loss plan. The surgeon inserts a narrow tube under your skin through tiny incisions, and then suctions out fat cells. It's most commonly used on the outer thighs and abdomen in women and on the sides or "love handles" in men.

Though liposuction has improved to allow surgeons to remove several pounds during one procedure, the surgery isn't a treatment for obesity. Liposuction is a body-shaping procedure for people of normal or near-normal weight who have problem spots — specific deposits of fat that don't go away despite a healthy diet and exercise.

People with certain weight-related medical conditions, including diabetes and heart disease, are at increased risk of complications from liposuction.

Recipes you can rely on

Here are recipes for some of the foods included in the 1,200-calorie and 1,400-calorie daily menus you'll find in Chapter 7 (see pages 94-101). You'll find additional recipes in our "Color guide to healthy eating" (see pages C7-C16). All of the recipes in this book are from our award-winning *Mayo Clinic/Williams-Sonoma Cookbook.*

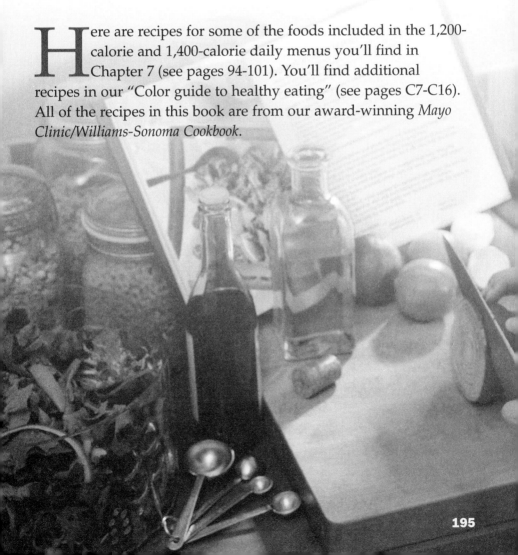

Sunshine juice blend

Wheat germ, the embryo of the wheat kernel, which is separated during milling, abounds in fiber. The strawberries and peaches add more fiber plus vitamin C, making this fruit-filled drink a wonderful way to start the day or finish a meal.

SERVES: 2 **PREPARATION:** 5 minutes

2 cups (8 oz/250 g) hulled fresh strawberries
1 peach, peeled, pitted, and coarsely chopped
1/2 cup (4 fl oz/125 mL) fat-free milk
2 tablespoons wheat germ
1 tablespoon honey
3 ice cubes

- In a blender, combine the strawberries, peach, milk, wheat germ, honey, and ice cubes. Blend until smooth, about 20 seconds.
- To serve, divide between glasses.

Provençal chicken and fennel

The braised combination of chicken breasts, fennel, tomatoes, and garlic, accented by a fragrant hint of grated orange zest, brings to mind a casual supper you might enjoy in the south of France. Serve with mashed potatoes.

SERVES: 6 **PREPARATION:** 25 minutes   **COOKING:** 30 minutes

6 small fennel bulbs, 3 lb (1.5 kg) total, trimmed
2 tomatoes, diced or 14 1/2 oz (455 g) canned diced tomatoes, drained
1/4 cup (2 fl oz/60 mL) dry white wine
1 tablespoon grated orange zest (peel)
3 garlic cloves, minced
2 teaspoons balsamic vinegar
1/8 teaspoon red pepper flakes
6 skinless, bone-in chicken breast halves, 5 oz (155 g) each, trimmed of visible fat
2 tablespoons chopped fresh flat-leaf (Italian) parsley

- Cut each fennel bulb in half lengthwise through the base. Cut each half into 4 wedges.
- In a large nonstick frying pan, combine the tomatoes, wine, orange zest (grated peel), garlic, vinegar, and pepper flakes. Cook

over medium heat, stirring occasionally, until the mixture comes to a boil. Reduce heat to medium-low.

- Arrange the chicken and fennel over the tomato mixture, spooning a bit of the sauce over them. Cover and cook until the chicken is opaque throughout and the fennel is tender, about 25 minutes. Using a slotted spoon, transfer the chicken and vegetables to a warmed platter.
- Increase heat to high and cook the sauce, stirring occasionally, until it has thickened slightly, about 5 minutes. Spoon the sauce over the chicken and vegetables and sprinkle with the parsley.
- To serve, divide among individual plates.

Summer savory spinach frittata

An open-faced omelet is a wonderful opportunity to try cholesterol-free, pasteurized egg product in place of 6 eggs. Either 5 cups (5 oz/155 g) of fresh spinach leaves, steamed, or 10 oz (315 g) frozen spinach, thawed, will yield the right amount of vegetable.

SERVES: 6 **PREPARATION:** 15 minutes **COOKING:** 20 minutes

1 1/2 cups (12 fl oz/375 mL) pasteurized egg product
2 tablespoons chopped fresh summer savory or 2 teaspoons dried summer savory
1 tablespoon water
1 tablespoon olive oil
1 cup (8 oz/250 g) cooked, chopped spinach
2 leeks, thinly sliced, including green portions
3/4 cup (3 1/2 oz/105 g) cooked peas or thawed frozen peas
1/2 teaspoon ground pepper
1/4 cup (1 oz/30 g) grated Gruyère or Swiss cheese
1/4 cup (1 oz/30 g) finely diced yellow or red bell pepper (capsicum)

- In a bowl, whisk together the egg product, summer savory, and water.
- In a large nonstick frying pan over medium heat, heat the oil. Add the spinach, leeks, peas, and pepper. Cook, stirring frequently, until the leeks are tender, about 10 minutes. Transfer to a bowl.
- To prevent the mixture from sticking, wipe the frying pan clean, then coat it with nonstick cooking spray. Return to medium heat. Put the vegetables back in the pan and pat them into an even

layer. Pour in the egg mixture; don't worry if it doesn't quite cover the vegetables. Cook, shaking the pan occasionally to keep the frittata from sticking, until the eggs are set around the edges but soft and runny in the center, about 3 minutes.

• Sprinkle with the cheese and bell pepper. Cover and cook, continuing to shake the frying pan occasionally, until the eggs are completely set and the cheese is melted, about 3 minutes longer.

• To serve, cut into wedges. Serve hot, warm, or cold.

Wild rice-and-chicken salad

Introducing fruit juice into a salad dressing adds enhanced flavor and texture without fat. Try substituting other juices or nectars for the pineapple juice called for here. Orange juice also marries well with the tastes of both the chicken breast and the wild rice.

SERVES: 6   **PREPARATION:** 20 minutes

1/4 cup (2 fl oz/60 mL) pineapple juice
11/2 tablespoons white wine vinegar
1 tablespoon Dijon mustard
3 garlic cloves, crushed with a garlic press
1/2 teaspoon ground pepper
11/2 tablespoons olive oil
6 cups (32 oz/1 kg) cooked, cold wild rice
3 cups (1 lb/500 g) cooked, shredded chicken breast meat
1 red bell pepper (capsicum), stemmed, seeded, and cut into 1/2-inch
    (12 mm) squares
6 green (spring) onions, thinly sliced, including green portions
1/2 cup (1/3 oz/10 g) chopped fresh basil
11/2 tablespoons capers, drained
3 cups (41/2 oz/140 g) chopped romaine lettuce

• In a large bowl, whisk together the pineapple juice, vinegar, mustard, garlic, and pepper. Add the olive oil and whisk until well blended.

• Add the wild rice, chicken, bell pepper, green onions, basil, and capers. Stir and toss to coat well with the dressing. Add the lettuce and toss to mix well.

• To serve, divide among individual plates.

Thai-style mushroom-and-tofu stir-fry

In this dish, the rich textures of mushrooms and tofu are highlighted by the savory flavors of peanut butter and sesame oil. Joined with crisp snow peas and water chestnuts, they make a hearty Asian-inspired main dish. Serve with steamed brown or white rice.

SERVES: 6   **PREPARATION:** 25 minutes   **COOKING:** 10 minutes

1/4 cup (2 oz/60 g) creamy reduced-fat peanut butter
2 tablespoons reduced-sodium soy sauce
2 tablespoons lime juice
1/3 cup (3 fl oz/80 mL) water
2 teaspoons sesame oil
2 teaspoons cornstarch (corn flour)
1/2 teaspoon red pepper flakes
12 oz (375 g) oyster mushrooms, sliced
1/2 lb (250 g) snow peas (mangetouts), ends trimmed and strings pulled
8 oz (250 g) canned sliced water chestnuts, rinsed and drained
1 lb (500 g) firm tofu, cut into 1/2-inch (12-mm) cubes
1/2 cup (2/3 oz/20 g) chopped cilantro (fresh coriander)

- In a small bowl, whisk together the peanut butter, soy sauce, and lime juice until smooth. Add the water, sesame oil, cornstarch, and pepper flakes and whisk until blended.
- Coat a nonstick wok or a large nonstick frying pan with non-stick cooking spray and heat over high heat. Add the mushrooms and stir-fry until lightly browned, about 4 minutes. Add the snow peas and continue stir-frying until the peas are tender-crisp, 2–3 minutes.
- Add the peanut butter mixture, water chestnuts and tofu, and stir-fry until the sauce thickens slightly, about 1 minute.
- To serve, transfer to a bowl. Sprinkle with the cilantro.

Gingered carrot soup

Because carrots are available year-round, this soup is designed to suit every season. In cold weather, serve it steaming hot as a starter whose ginger aroma will entice diners. In warm weather, serve it chilled as a refreshing beverage.

SERVES: 6 **PREPARATION:** 15 minutes + 4 hours if chilling **COOKING:** 25 minutes
1 tablespoon olive oil
6 large carrots, peeled and cut into chunks
1 onion, thinly sliced
2 celery stalks, thinly sliced
3 tablespoons chopped celery leaves
2 cups (16 fl oz/500 mL) water
2 cups (16 fl oz/500 mL) canned vegetable broth
1 slice whole-wheat (whole-meal) sandwich bread, torn into bits
1/4 cup (2 fl oz/60 mL) nonfat evaporated milk
1/2 cup (1/2 oz/15 g) thinly sliced green (spring) onion tops
2 tablespoons grated fresh ginger

- In a large saucepan over medium heat, heat the oil. Add the carrots, onion, celery, and celery leaves. Sauté for 5 minutes.
- Stir in the water, broth, and bread. Increase heat to high and bring to a boil.
- Reduce heat to low, cover, and simmer until the carrots are tender, about 20 minutes.
- Transfer the soup — in batches, if necessary — to a blender or food processor and purée until smooth.
- To serve hot, return the soup to the saucepan and stir in the milk and green onions. Reheat for a moment over low heat, not letting the soup boil, then stir in the ginger. Ladle into individual bowls.
- To serve cold, pour into a large bowl and stir in the milk, green onions, and ginger. Cool to room temperature, then cover and refrigerate until chilled thoroughly, at least 4 hours or up to 3 days. Ladle into mugs.

Recipes reprinted from *The Mayo Clinic | Williams-Sonoma Cookbook* with permission of Weldon Owen, Inc. The book is available at bookstores, Williams-Sonoma stores and mail order (see page 210 for ordering information).

Index

A

Acetaminophen, 109
Activity, physical, 105–124
    aches and pains, 109
    and arthritis, 110–111
    and coronary artery disease,
        109–110
    and diabetes, 110
    exercise programs, 115–124
    and extreme obesity, 111
    getting children involved,
        111–113
    guidelines, 24–25, 106–107
    low-intensity activities, 108
    and osteoporosis, 110
Acutrim, 182
Adult-onset diabetes. *See also*
        Type 2 diabetes mellitus
Aerobic dance, 119
Aerobic exercise, 116–119
    calories burned, 117
    target heart rate, 122
Affirmations, positive, 141–142
Age and body fat, 8, 9
Alcohol consumption
    and beer, 36
    and excess calories, 26, 73
    and syndrome X, 36
    calories per gram, 26
American vs. Chinese dietary
        habits, 25
Anorexia nervosa, 35
Antidepressants, 28
Apnea, sleep, 32
Appetite suppressants, 182

Apples and pears, 34
Arthritis, 110–111
Atkins diet, 163
Attitudes and beliefs, 7, 125–145,
        148–149

B

Baking, 68
Barley, 50
Basil, 69
Bay leaf, 69
Beef, lean cuts, 54
Beer and alcohol drinking, 36
Behavior modification chain,
        136, 155–156
Benefits of weight loss, 5, 33, 37
Beverly Hills diet, 167
Bicycling, 119
Blood type diet, 167–168
Body fat
    apple vs. pear shape, 34
    changes with age, 8, 9
    in healthy adults, 15–16
Body mass index (BMI)
    chart, 17
    formula, 17
    interactive calculator, 18
Braising food, 68
Bread, 85–86
Broccoli in spicy orange sauce,
        C9
Broiling food, 68
Bulgur, 50
Bulimia nervosa, 35

C

Cabbage soup diet, 168
Caffeine and weight loss, 182
Calories
  and excess sugar
    consumption, 9
  energy density, 58
  and energy sources, 26
  expended during exercise,
    117
  to gain or lose a pound, 27
  recommended daily, 79–80
  volume of food, 9–11, 78
Cancer and overweight, 33
Caraway, 69
Carbohydrates
  best choices and serving
    sizes, 85–86, C5
  calories per gram, 26
  complex, 55
  dietary recommendations, 56
  food group, 61
  low-carbohydrate diets, 56
  nutritional need for, 55
  simple, 55
  types and sources, 55, 57
Changing habits, 132–138, 146–149
  forming good habits, 146-149
  preparation for, 130–138
  stages, 42
Chervil, 69
Children and activity planning,
    111–113
Chili powder, 69
Chinese vs. American dietary
    habits, 25
Chitosan, 181
Chocolate pudding pie, C16
Cholesterol
  dietary sources, 53, 57
  HDL, 30
Cilantro, 71
CitraLean, 181

CitriMax, 181
Citrus Slim Gum, 181
Cleaning your plate, 40–41, 135
Complex carbohydrates, 55
Cooking and preparation tips.
    See also Recipes
  fruits, 60
  general, 67–72
  glossary of cooking methods,
    68
  legumes, 62
  modifying recipes, 69, 70
  safe food handling, 67
  vegetables, 59
Cooking Light, 139
Coriander, 71
Coronary artery disease, 31,
    109–110
Corticosteroids, 28
Cravings, 138–139, 154
Cumin, 71

D

Dairy foods, 61–62
DASH diet, 91
Depression, 141, 172
Deprivation, feelings, 138–139
Desserts
  best choices, 134
  weekly allowance, 88–89
Dexatrim, 182
Diabetes (type 2), 31, 110
Diet plans
  Atkins diet, 163
  commercial groups, 169–172
  fad diets, 165–168
  high protein/low
    carbohydrate, 163
  low-calorie liquid diets,
    162–163
  low-calorie solid-food diets,
    163–165
  Overeaters Anonymous, 172

Diet plans — cont.
prepared-food plans, 168–169
questions to ask, 164, 170
Sugar Busters, 161, 165
TOPS Club, Inc., 156, 171
The Zone, 161, 164–165
Weight Watchers, 156,
170–171
Diet vs. weight-loss diet, 23
"Dieter's attitude," 7, 8, 157
"Dieting" vs. healthy eating,
6–7, 43
Dietitians (registered), 44, 186
Dill, 71
Dining record, 92–93
Discrimination against the
overweight, 5
Drugs. *See also* Medications
Dumping syndrome, 185
Duodenum, 191

E
Eating disorders, 35
Eating late at night, 40, 152
Eating mindfully, 132–133
Eating out, 22, 57, 72–74
Eicosanoids, 164–165
Elliptical cross-training machine,
119–120
Energy balance, 26–27
Energy density of foods, 58,
61, 78
Ephedrine, 180–181
Excuses, 41–42
Exercise, physical. *See also*
Activity, physical.
aerobic, 116–119
calories burned during, 117
flexibility and stretching,
121–122
Perceived Exertion Scale, 118
recording activities, 122, 124
strength and balance,
120–121

Exercise, physical — cont.
structured programs, 113–114
target heart rate, 124
vs. activity, 23–25, 105-106
warning signs, 122

F
Fad diets, 165-168
Family activities, 111–113
Family medical history, 8,
21–22, 36
Fats and oils, 87-88
best choices and serving
sizes, 88, C5
calories per gram, 26
daily recommendations, 65
food group, 62-63
nutritional need for, 52
reduced-fat foods, 52, 54
substitutions in recipes, 70
types, 53
Fat cells, 3, 29
Favorite foods, 40, 153–156
Fen-phen, 177
Fiber
and energy density, 78
health benefits, 55–56
Fidgeting, 107
Fitness magazines, 45
5-HTP (5-hydroxytryptophan),
182
Flexibility and stretching,
121–122
Food cravings, 138-139, 154
Food groups, 58–64
Food journal, 129–130
Food labels, 65–66
Food record, 90-93
Food safety, 67
Food triggers, 40–41, 90, 132
Fruits
best choices and serving
sizes, 84–85, C4
types, 60

G

Gaining weight
  and low-fat foods, 54
  and medications, 28
  and pregnancy, 28
  and smoking cessation, 27
Gallstones, 32
Gastric banding, 189
Gastric bypass, 191–192
Gastric partitioning (stapling),
  189
Genetics, 8, 21–22, 36
Getting started
  adding activity to your life,
    108
  are you ready?, 10–11
  changing habits, 132–138,
    146–149
  check with your doctor, 115
  making healthful food
    choices, 82–89
  preparing to change, 42–44
  setting goals, 44–45, 79-80,
    149–150
Ginger, 71
Goal-setting, 45–46, 79, 149–150
Good habits, forming, 146–149
Grapefruit diet, 166–167
Grilling food, 68

H

Habits, changing, 132–138,
  146–149
HCA (hydroxycitric acid), 181
HDL cholesterol, 30
Health clubs, 113–114
Health magazines, 45
Healthy eating, 49–74, C1–C5
Healthy weight
  body mass index (BMI), 16, 17
  self-assessment, 34, 36–37
  success statistics, 160
Heart attack during exercise, 109

Heart failure and sleep apnea,
  32
Herbal dietary supplements,
  180–183
Herbs and spices, 69, 71–72
Heredity, 8, 21–22, 36
Hernia after surgery, 193
High blood pressure
  (hypertension), 30
High fiber, 55
High-protein diets
  health risks of, 57, 163
  myths, 56
Home exercise equipment,
  114–115
Hydroxycitic acid, 181
Hypertension (high blood
  pressure), 30
Hyssop, 71

I

Insulin resistance, 56–57
Ischemic stroke, 31–32

J

Jejunoileal bypass, 188–189
Jejunum, 191
Jenny Craig, 169
Jogging, 117–119

K

Kale, 50
Kasha, 50
Kiwi fruit, 50

L

Late-night snacking, 40, 152
Laxatives, 182
LEARN behavior programs,
  136, 139, 155
Legumes, 62
Lifespan and excess weight, 33
Lifestyle factors, 3, 25

"Light" foods, 66
Liposuction, 194
Liquid diets, 162–163
Low-carbohydrate diets, risks of, 57
Low-fat foods
 lean meat, 54
Low-intensity activities, 108

M

Mace, 71
Magazines, fitness and health, 45
Mango, 51
Marjoram, 71
"Mayo Clinic Diet myth," 103
Mayo Clinic Healthy Weight Pyramid
 chart and guidelines, C1–C3
 daily dining record, 92–93
 DASH diet, 91
 features, 79
 food groups, 58–64
 food recommendations, C4-C5
 and USDA Dietary Guidelines, 104
Mayo Clinic Internet home page, 12. *See also* Web site address.
Mayo Clinic/Williams-Sonoma Cookbook, 195
Meat
 cooking and preparation tips, 67–68
 lean cuts, 54
Medications, 175–183. *See also* OTC dietary supplements, Herbal dietary supplements.
 and weight gain, 28
 appetite suppressants, 182
 corticosteroids, 28
 fen-phen, 177
 5-HTP (5-hydroxytryptophan), 182

Medications — cont.
 hydroxycitric acid (HCA), 181
 laxatives, 182
 Meridia (sibutramine), 178–179
 phentermine, 177
 phenylpropanolamine hydrochloride, 182
 pyruvate, 183
 Saint John's wort, 182
 tricyclic antidepressants, 28
 when appropriate, 176
 Xenical (orlistat), 179–180
Medifast, 162
Mediterranean-style diet, 102
Menu planning, 94–101, 102, 133
Meridia (sibutramine), 178–179
Metab-O-LITE, 180
Metabolic disorders, 8
Metabolife, 180–181
MetaboMax, 180
Milk, 63
Monounsaturated fat, 53, 63
Motivation, 10–11, 43, 127–128, 141–142
Muscle vs. fat, 8

N

NEAT (nonexercise activity thermogenesis), 107
Neck size and sleep apnea, 32
NutriSystem, 169
Nutrition
 carbohydrate recommendations, 54-57
 food groups, 58–64
 food labels, 65–66
 and the Mayo Clinic Healthy Weight Pyramid, 79, 82
 reduced-fat foods, 54
 variety in diet, 50
 vitamin supplements, 82
 and weight-loss surgery, 192

O

Obesity
  and activity planning, 111
  causes, 21–28
  defined, 15, 16-17
  health risks, 4, 29–33
  incidence in United States, 5
  and water retention, 30
Oils. *See also* Fats and oils
Optifast, 162
orlistat (Xenical), 179-180
Osteoarthritis, 32
Osteoporosis, 110
Overeaters Anonymous, 172
Overeating, 151, 153
Over-the-counter (OTC) dietary
    supplements, 180-183
Overweight. *See also* Obesity
  defined, 15-17
  health risks, 4, 29–33
  incidence in United States, 3, 5

P

Pennsylvania State University,
    58, 78
Perceived Exertion Scale, 118
Phytochemicals, 57
Planning ahead, 46
Poaching food, 68
Polyunsaturated fat, 53
Portion size
  measuring, 57, C5
  reducing, 41, 57
Pregnancy and weight gain, 28
Prepared-food diet plans,
    168–169
Problem-solving, 151–153
Processed foods, 23
Protein
  best choices and serving
      sizes, 87, C5
  calories per gram, 26
  nutritional need for, 61

Protein — cont.
  protein and dairy food
      group, 61–63
Pyloric valve, 187
Pyruvate, 183

R

Recipe sources, 45, 139, 195
Recipes
  broccoli in spicy orange
      sauce, C9
  chocolate pudding pie, C16
  gingered carrot soup,
      199–200
  hearty grain-filled peppers,
      C13
  how to modify, 70
  minted Mediterranean fruit
      mix, C7
  poached salmon with melon
      salsa, C15
  Provençal chicken and
      fennel, 196–197
  sesame asparagus-and-carrot
      stir-fry, C11
  summer savory spinach
      frittata, 197–198
  sunshine juice blend, 196
  Thai-style mushroom-and-
      tofu stir-fry, 199
  wild rice-and-chicken salad,
      198
Reduced-fat foods, 54
Refined vs. whole grain foods, 85
Restaurant meals, 22, 57–58,
    72–74
Risks of excess weight, 4, 29–34
Roasting foods, 68
Rosemary, 71

S

Saffron, 72
Sage, 72

Satiety (feeling full), 78
Saturated fat, 53
Sautéing, 68
Sedentary lifestyle, defined, 24
Self-control vs. willpower,
    153–156
Serving, number of, 81, C4
Sesame asparagus and carrot
    stir-fry, C11
Setbacks, 112, 131–132, 145–160
Shape magazine, 45
Shopping tips
    food labels, 65–66
    fruits, 60
    general, 64–67
    lean beef cuts, 54
    legumes, 62
    reduced-fat foods, 54
    vegetables, 59
    whole grains, 61
sibutramine (Merida), 178-179
Simple carbohydrates, 55
Ski machines, 119
Sleep apnea, 32–33
Slim-Fast, 162–163
Small-bowel bypass, 188–189
Smoking cigarettes
    and metabolic rate, 27–28
    quitting and weight gain, 28
Sodium
    in canned vegetables, 59
    and excess weight, 30
Soy
    tempeh, 51
    textured soy protein, 51
    tofu, 51
Spices and herbs, 69, 71–72
Saint John's wort, 182
Starches, 55
Starting calorie level, 80
Steaming food, 68
Stir-frying food, 68
Strength and balance training,
    120–121

Stroke, ischemic, 31–32
Substitutions in recipes, 70
Success statistics, 160
Sugar Busters, 165
Sugar consumption, 9, 22–23, 89
Support for changing habits,
    136, 156–157
Surgery for weight loss, 185–194
    adjustments, 193
    dietitians, 186
    gastric stapling, 189
    gastric bypass, 191–192
    gastric partitioning
        (stapling), 189
    psychologists, 186
    side effects, 192–193
    small-bowel bypass, 188–189
    vertical-banded gastroplasty,
        190–191
    when needed, 186–187
        Sweets food group
    best choices, 134
    daily allowance, 88–89
    defined, 63
    weekly allowance, 88
Swimming, 119
Syndrome X, 34, 36

T
Target heart rate for exercise,
    122
Tarragon, 72
Television and overeating, 40
Tempeh, 51
Textured soy protein, 51
Thyme, 72
Tofu, 51
TOPS Club, 156, 171
Trans fat, 53
Triglycerides, 30–31
Tylenol (acetaminophen), 109
Type 2 diabetes mellitus, 31

U

Underweight and BMI
defined, 19
University of Alabama at
Birmingham, 58, 78, 79

V

Variety in diet, 50–51
Vegetables
best choices and serving
sizes, 83–84, C4
types, 59–60
Vegetarian Times magazine, 45
Vertical-banded gastroplasty,
190–191
Visualization, 46
Vitamin supplements, 82, 183
VLCDs (very-low-calorie liquid-
based diets), 162–163

W

Waist measurement and health
risks, 18
Walking, 116–117
Walking magazine, 45
Water retention, 30
Web site addresses
LEARN behavior programs,
136
Mayo Clinic Internet home
page, 12
Weight gain
and fad diets, 148
and low-fat foods, 54
and medications, 28
and pregnancy, 28
and smoking cessation, 27
Weight-lifting, 120–121
Weight loss. *See also* Diet plans
benefits, 5, 33, 37
daily calories recommended,
80
evaluating programs, 170

Weight loss — cont.
fad diets, 165–168
food record, 90–93
importance of activity,
105–124
menus, 94–101
motivation, 10–11, 43,
127–128, 141–142
and nutritional needs, 82-88
recommended rate, 10–11
risks of rapid, 32
serving recommendations, 81
success statistics, 160
surgery, 185–194
wrong reasons for, 6
Weight Watchers, 156, 170-171
Whole grains, 61, 85-86
Willpower vs. self-control,
153–156

X

Xenical (orlistat), 179–180

Z

Zone, The, 164–165

MAYO CLINIC ON HEALTH

Arthritis

Chronic Pain

Depression

Digestive Health

Healthy Aging

Healthy Weight

High Blood Pressure

Managing Diabetes

Prostate Health

Vision